AF172545

Measurement and Analysis in Transforming Healthcare Delivery

Harry C. Sax

Editor

Measurement and Analysis in Transforming Healthcare Delivery

Volume 2: Practical Applications
to Engage and Align Providers
and Consumers

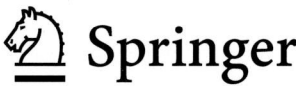 Springer

Editor
Harry C. Sax
Department of Surgery
Cedars Sinai Medical Center
Los Angeles, CA, USA

ISBN 978-3-319-46220-2   ISBN 978-3-319-46222-6   (eBook)
DOI 10.1007/978-3-319-46222-6

Library of Congress Control Number: 2016943088

© Springer International Publishing Switzerland 2017
This work is subject to copyright. All rights are reserved by the Publisher, whether the whole or part of the material is concerned, specifically the rights of translation, reprinting, reuse of illustrations, recitation, broadcasting, reproduction on microfilms or in any other physical way, and transmission or information storage and retrieval, electronic adaptation, computer software, or by similar or dissimilar methodology now known or hereafter developed.
The use of general descriptive names, registered names, trademarks, service marks, etc. in this publication does not imply, even in the absence of a specific statement, that such names are exempt from the relevant protective laws and regulations and therefore free for general use.
The publisher, the authors and the editors are safe to assume that the advice and information in this book are believed to be true and accurate at the date of publication. Neither the publisher nor the authors or the editors give a warranty, express or implied, with respect to the material contained herein or for any errors or omissions that may have been made.

Printed on acid-free paper

This Springer imprint is published by Springer Nature
The registered company is Springer International Publishing AG
The registered company address is: Gewerbestrasse 11, 6330 Cham, Switzerland

To my children, Ben, Adam and Rachel; it is for their generation, and those that follow, that we have to get healthcare right

Preface

To say there is uncertainty in healthcare is an understatement. To suggest that change is needed is obvious. How we do it, and how we measure the effectiveness of those interventions is where the real challenge lies.

In my own career as an academic surgeon, I have at times been frustrated by multiple forces working at crossed purposes. Incentives are misaligned, outcomes measures do not fully reflect the complexity of the process, and patients are often overwhelmed with options. Healthcare executives and clinicians try to provide patient-centric care in a heavily regulated and litigious environment. Yet despite these challenges, organizations have emerged that are achieving the Institute of Healthcare Improvement "Triple Aim" of improving the patient experience of care, improving the health of populations, and reducing the per capita cost of healthcare. This book hopes to capture the lessons learned by those successes and give the reader tools and ideas relevant for their own situation.

Although this volume has an emphasis on American healthcare delivery, we have drawn from experts familiar with alternative models, including single payer systems. We strove to provide the reader with clear definitions of quality, efficiency, financial, and appropriateness measures. Chapters focusing on leading change and motivating others may provide ideas that are applicable in one's own organization. We hope to capture lessons learned from the past to reduce the uncertainty of the future.

Los Angeles, CA   Harry C. Sax

Acknowledgments

I have been fortunate to have had mentors who helped organize my thinking and taught by example. Some were supervisors, and many were colleagues. During residency at the University of Cincinnati, my Chairman, Dr. Josef Fischer, insisted that excellence was expected and everything else needed an explanation. He provided me my first understanding of the business concepts of medical delivery and research. Dr. Seymour Schwartz, at the University of Rochester, gave me my first job in 1989. He was the ultimate Renaissance man and emphasized the humanistic aspects of leadership. My colleagues at The Miriam Hospital and Brown University helped me round out my understanding of medical staff functioning, collaboration with the community, and how to interface with governmental agencies. We took risks with data transparency, individual practitioner report cards, and integration of new technology. The chance to go back to school at age 52 at the Harvard Masters in Health Care Management Program was energizing and gave me new tools and insights. As good as the professors were, the 17 other physicians from around the world were my everyday teachers. We spent more than a few nights in the hotel lobby, figuring out solutions to case studies…. and our lives. My current Chair at Cedars-Sinai, Dr. Bruce Gewertz, exemplifies leadership in all he does, with a combination of pragmatism, humor, and a deep understanding of people. He and the former Chair of Medicine, Dr. Glenn Braunstein, were gracious in creating a new position for me when I was transitioning my career to focus on healthcare management, quality, and safety.

Barbara Lopez-Lucio and her colleagues at Springer gently pushed to keep me on track with this book and provided alternatives when we hit roadblocks. It has been a pleasure to work with them.

Contents

Contributors

Charles E. Coffey Jr., M.D., M.S., F.H.M., F.A.C.P. Los Angeles County + University of Southern California Medical Center, Los Angeles, CA, USA

Yishay Falick, M.D., M.B.A. Department of Medical Affairs, Ministry of Health, Jerusalem, Israel

Bruce L. Gewertz, M.D. Department of Surgery, Cedars-Sinai Medical Center, Los Angeles, CA, USA

Thomas R. Graf, M.D. The Chartis Group, Pine Grove, PA, USA

Victoria G. Hines, M.H.A. University of Rochester Medical Faculty Group, University of Rochester Medical Center, Rochester, NY, USA

Monica Jain, M.D. Department of Surgery, Cedars-Sinai Medical Center, Los Angeles, CA, USA

Brett McCone, B.A., M.H.A. Department of Rate Setting, Maryland Hospital Association, Elkridge, MD, USA

David Norris, B.S-.C.S. MD Insider, Santa Monica, CA, USA

Teryl K. Nuckols, M.D., M.S.H.S. Department of Medicine, Cedars Sinai Medical Center, Los Angeles, CA, USA

Michael F. Rotondo, M.D., F.A.C.S. University of Rochester Medical Faculty Group, University of Rochester Medical Center, Rochester, NY, USA

Harry C. Sax, M.D., F.A.C.S., F.A.C.H.E. Department of Surgery, Cedars Sinai Medical Center, Los Angeles, CA, USA

Steven R. Sosland, M.B.A., B.S. Office of People Development, University of North Texas Health Science Center, Fort Worth, TX, USA

Glenn D. Steele Jr., M.D., Ph.D. xG Health Solutions, Danville, PA, USA

Michael R. Williams, D.O., M.D., M.B.A. University of North Texas Health Science Center, Fort Worth, TX, USA

Eyal Zimlichman, M.D., M.Sc. Central Management, Sheba Medical Center, Ramat Gan, Israel

Chapter 1
Healthcare Transformation: What Are the Challenges?

Harry C. Sax

Healing is a matter of time, but it is also a matter of opportunity.

Hippocrates

Overview

With the unprecedented expansion of both capability and cost, medicine stands at a crossroads—we have the ability to correct defects at the cellular level, yet cannot deliver consistent, evidence-based, appropriate care to broad segments of society. In the United States, healthcare expenditures approach 18 % of Gross Domestic Product, yet measured outcomes in areas such as infant mortality, and access to care are not commensurate with the resources consumed [1]. Headlines suggest we are killing over 100,000 patients a year through medical error, yet mandated process measures with incentives and penalties have not significantly reduced this number [2, 3]. To address these challenges, we must understand the current state, measure relevant data, and understand interactions of multiple stakeholders to align a cohesive response.

This volume is a complement to Dr. Fabri's excellent treatise on the mechanics of measurement. His in-depth analysis of statistical methods clearly outlines the potential and the limitations of quantitative data. He emphasizes that correlation may not be causation, and that the application of big data to the individual patient is different from that of populations. With this as the base, we will focus on what to measure in the real world, and how to translate those findings into actionable items.

H.C. Sax, M.D., F.A.C.S., F.A.C.H.E. (✉)
Department of Surgery, Cedars Sinai Medical Center, 8700 Beverly Blvd;
NT 8215, Los Angeles, CA 90048, USA
e-mail: Harry.Sax@cshs.org

© Springer International Publishing Switzerland 2017
H.C. Sax (ed.), *Measurement and Analysis in Transforming Healthcare Delivery*, DOI 10.1007/978-3-319-46222-6_1

The initial chapters outline both quantitative and qualitative measures to aid in the system design and benchmarking necessary for successful transformation. The outcomes of single payer systems are examined as many analogies can be drawn to the move away from fee for service and to global budgeting. Finally, experienced leaders will share how they combined data with an understanding of human motivation to achieve remarkable results.

We open focusing on specific definitions of hospital performance. Although increasing amounts of care are delivered outside of the acute hospital setting, it is nonetheless critical to understand how resources flow and are consumed, as well as the quality of what is delivered. From a pubic planning perspective, it is advantageous to reduce duplication of services without impacting access. Further, Birkmeyer and others have shown a clear relationship between hospital volumes for high index procedures and better outcomes [4]. McCone's chapter shares perspectives from the Maryland Hospital Association's experience with a statewide All Payer Model and has an excellent description of how costs are allocated in an acute care setting. For any organization to survive, expand, and meet its missions, margins are required. As payment models change, the way we approach this equation must adapt.

The success of any delivery system is highly dependent on the health care providers within it. Norris describes the mechanism for developing and validating individual physician score cards, a highly sensitive issue among doctors. The key to the acceptance of a performance-based assessment is clear risk adjustment and holding individuals responsible only for those things over which they truly have control. Inherent to any assessment of performance is the issue of transparency. Over 20 years ago, New York State published the individual outcomes of cardiac surgeons and the hospitals in which they worked. The methodology included risk adjustment and also controlled for volume. The results were as one would expect—after a period of criticizing methodology—a gradual acceptance ensued. Poorly performing programs either improved or closed, well-performing institutions were encouraged to share their best practices, referrals shifted, and overall results were significantly enhanced [5]. With the Internet, formal and informal rating systems abound, but validation of the results and methodology is variable. For those who are rated, there is a tendency to advertise and celebrate those reports that make one look good and dismiss those that do not as measuring the wrong things. The techniques described in this chapter will help in "rating the raters."

How well we deliver care is one component of transformation—another is whether the care we deliver is appropriate both for the patient and for those that must decide how to allocate fixed resources. This is not to imply that care is being "rationed." Rather it is to recognize that not all care delivers the best overall outcome for the patient, given the risks, benefits, and costs. In their examination of appropriateness, Coffey and Nuckols tackle this tricky question and give practical example of how organizations have integrated these guidelines for the benefit of the patient. Guidelines are necessary but not sufficient. A key component remains open discussions between the patient and their clinician in developing plans of care. This is especially acute at the end of life when family dynamics often come into play.

Perhaps most telling is physicians' own choices for their care at the end of life compared to the more aggressive ones they recommend for their patients [6].

In addition to examining individual performance, entire groups of physicians must be aligned to deliver integrated care. Hines and Rotondo discuss the development of a multidisciplinary medical staff group at the University of Rochester. Academic medical centers have different missions than community hospitals or smaller primary care groups. Although there is the tendency to feel that the best way to influence clinicians is to employ them, this is not necessarily the case. Multiple different methods of risk and gain sharing are available, and one size does not necessarily fit all. It is encouraging that legislation, such as the Comprehensive Joint Replacement initiative, increases the ability for hospitals and practitioners to share risk and gain—something that was previously inhibited by Stark Regulations [7].

Success in the emerging healthcare landscape will require all of the tools noted earlier, combined with seamless vertical and horizontal integration. There are numerous examples of success in this realm; one of the most cited is the Geisinger system. Graf and Steele describe their journey of bringing together multiple stakeholders for the benefit of the patient. What is most striking is that full-time employment was not a prerequisite to success. Instead, they led a relentless focus on quality, best practices, and data-driven transparent outcomes. Successful programs that were initially developed for patients covered by the Geisinger Insurance product were scaled and opened to broader groups, including at-risk populations. The patient-centered focus included a guaranteed price for cardiac surgery including follow-up, as well as the offer to refund patients' costs, if they were not satisfied with their care. Clinicians seek to be part of the system [8].

In theory, having accurate data, validated clinical pathways, well trained healthcare providers, and adequate infrastructure should yield consistent, high-quality outcomes. Yet why is it that many heavily resourced organizations do not reach their full potential, and others that struggle in poor economic circumstances can flourish? The key is leadership setting a clear vision and influencing others to follow their own "True North." Williams and Sosland relate their experience in two organizations—Hill Country Memorial Hospital (HCMH) and the University of North Texas Health Science Center (UNTHSC). HCMH is a critical access hospital in Fredericksburg, Texas. It was struggling for survival, had poor outcomes, low patient satisfaction, and a disengaged medical staff. A sentinel event further galvanized the community. Leadership responded by focusing on inherent core values, a willingness to be relentless in open examination of opportunities, and creating a culture of both accountability and support. Their chapter described a transformation from a hospital near death to a Baldrige award winner. Similar challenges were encountered at UNTHSC, an emerging academic medical center in the highly competitive environment of the Dallas Fort Worth metroplex. What becomes apparent is that driving the transformation of an organization leads to personal growth as well.

Virtually every other developed country has some form of a single payer system with near universal coverage for basic needs. Zimlichman and Falick, Israeli academic physicians who also have experience in the American system, focus on what works and what does not in a single payer system. Israel is a hybrid, with competing

HMOs, as well as a flourishing secondary market for those patients who wish to pay more to receive more. Further, Israel recognizes the importance of emerging health-care technologies and dedicates a specific portion of the budget to innovation. Similar to the United States, there are challenges with providing care to a large number of noncitizens from neighboring countries and territories.

Key Concepts

Although each of the chapters has a different focus, several key themes emerge:

- We must acknowledge that there will be variability in outcomes within a popula-tion and that standardization will reduce some, but not all of that variability.
- Although in Lake Woebegone, "all the children are above average" [9], it is sta-tistically impossible that every practitioner and system will function in the top 50%. We must find ways to assess accurately the skills of the practitioner and assure that they are working in systems that allow them to optimize those skills. Current dashboards provide some information, but attribution, risk adjustment, team based care, and the low incidence of key metrics such as mortality make it difficult to truly identify high- and low-performing physicians.
- All healthcare providers, and those that lead, must develop new sets of skills centered around the "softer" competencies—emotional intelligence, servant leadership, and adapting to the different motivators of multigenerational, multi-cultural workforces.
- We must understand that just because we *can* do something does not mean we *should* do something. The care we provide must be appropriate for the situa-tion—and this will vary based on age, physical condition, and patient prefer-ences. In America, we have difficulty discussing care at the end of life and the dying process. Even support of the dialog between physicians and their patients has been politicized into "Death Panels" [10].
- We must set reasonable expectations with patients and their families to avoid disappointment (and possible litigation). Other countries have created stream-lined arbitration panels, chaired by professionals, that can rapidly evaluate and compensate a patient harmed by error [11]. Defensive medicine and its associated costs are reduced. Physicians are still held accountable for true errors of commis-sion, but there is a stronger tendency toward Marx's "Just Culture" [12].
- We must recognize that physicians are motivated by multiple factors, one of the strongest of which is autonomy to make the best choices for and with their patients. Most of us were drawn to the field for the ability to make a difference in a patient's life, and to test and challenge ourselves. Definition of a physician's value by the number of work RVUs generated, or contribution margin to a ser-vice line, is a way to create a disengaged, if nonetheless busy, medical staff. Under new payment models, physicians will be incented *not* to provide certain types of care, and will need to be engaged in other ways that bring value.

- Although beyond the scope of this book, medical education with the significant monetary and time commitment it entails is creating a generation of physicians who will spend most of their careers trying to get out from under significant debt. The incentive to move to better paying subspecialties exacerbates the maldistribution of primary care practitioners [13]. New options for earlier tracking to desired specialties and broadened opportunities for financial support in exchange for public service may stem this trend. To make sure that physicians are doing what they are uniquely trained for, we must support non-MD providers practicing at the top of their license.
- Current payment systems are complex, disjointed, and fraught with misaligned incentives. The pressures to reduce length of stay and penalize readmissions come without clear resources for improving transitions of care. It is interesting that many single payer countries, with lower overall healthcare expenditures, have longer average inpatient lengths of stay [14, 15]. As the United States moves to more bundled payments and risk-based contracts, it will be vital to encourage innovative partnerships among all stakeholders. Although fee for service, per se, will become less prominent, natural market forces will continue to be in play and tiered levels of care will emerge.
- Finally, we must embrace the current tumult as our greatest opportunity to return to the core of why we care for our fellow man, both in sickness and in health; that we as a society are willing to use resources to maintain the vitality of our community and that we will strive to provide appropriate care, in the right setting, for the right reasons.

References

1. Organization for Economic Cooperation and Development. Healthcare share of GDP by country, 2016. Modern Healthcare. 2016. http://www.modernhealthcare.com/article/20160206/DATA/500035409.
2. Ingraham AM, Cohen ME, Bilimoria KY, Dimick JB, Richards KE, Raval MV, Fleisher LA, Hall BL, Ko CY. Association of surgical care improvement project infection-related process measure compliance with risk-adjusted outcomes: implications for quality measurement. J Am Coll Surg. 2010;211(6):705–14.
3. Altman DE, Clancy C, Blendon RJ. Improving patient safety—five years after the IOM report. N Engl J Med. 2004;351(20):2041–3.
4. Birkmeyer JD, Siewers AE, Finlayson EVA, et al. Hospital volume and surgical mortality in the United States. N Engl J Med. 2002;346:1128–37.
5. Thourani VH, Sarin EL. Influence of cardiac surgeon report cards on patient referral by cardiologists in New York state after 20 years of public reporting. Circ Cardiovasc Qual Outcomes. 2013;6(6):617–8.
6. Murray K. How doctors die. Saturday Evening Post; March/April 2013.
7. Center for Medicare and Medicaid Services. Comprehensive care for joint replacement. 2015. https://www.federalregister.gov/articles/2015/11/24/2015–29438/medicare-program-comprehensive-care-for-joint-replacement-payment-model-for-acute-care-hospitals. e pub 24 Nov 2015.
8. Ellison A. Geisinger's money-back guarantee is about more than refunds. Beckers Hospital Review. http://www.beckershospitalreview.com/finance/geisinger-s-money-back-guarantee-is-about-more-than-refunds.html. Accessed 9 Dec 2015.
9. Keillor G. Lake Woebegone days. New York: Penguin; 1986.

10. Nyhan B. Why the "death panel" myth wouldn't die: misinformation in the health care reform debate. Forum. 2010;18:1–24.
11. Gallagher TH, Waterman AD, Garbutt JM, Kapp JM, Chan DK, Dunagan WC, Fraser VJ, Levinson W. US and Canadian physicians' attitudes and experiences regarding disclosing errors to patients. Arch Intern Med. 2006;166(15):1605–11.
12. Frankel AS, Leonard MW, Dehham CR. Engagement: the tools to achieve high reliability. Health Serv Res. 2006;41(4 Pt 2):1690–709.
13. Phillips JP, Petterson SM, Bazemore AW, Phillips RL. A Retrospective analysis of the relationship between medical student debt and primary care practice in the United States. Ann Fam Med. 2014;12(6):542–9.
14. Centers for Disease Control. Hospital utilization (in non-Federal short stay hospitals). http://www.cdc.gov/nchs/fastats/hospital.htm. Updated 27 April 2016.
15. National Health Service. Length of stay—reducing length of stay. 2013. http://www.institute.nhs.uk/quality_and_service_improvement_tools/quality_and_service_improvement_tools/length_of_stay.html.

Chapter 2
Terminology and Applications: Hospital Performance Measures

Brett McCone

Introduction

Hospital performance measures are created and applied for a myriad of reasons. They range from purely financial—how much it costs to produce something, to purely clinical—the patient did or did not contract another condition before discharge. Inherent in the use of hospital performance measures is the desire to increase value. Health care value is defined as quality (output) divided by cost (input) [1]. To transform health care delivery, hospital performance measures should be viewed through the lens of value.

While cost and quality are often the basis of hospital performance measures, it is important to understand the context of hospital payment incentives. Most United States hospitals are subject to different payment incentives from Medicare, Medicaid, and commercial insurance, including Blue Cross plans, health maintenance organizations, etc. The payment incentives, particularly Medicare, can drive behavior that directly or indirectly affect hospital performance on any measure or series of measures. Maryland's All-Payer Demonstration Model is a unique exception that attempts to align incentives across all payers and is worth exploring further.

In addition to hospital payment incentives, to successfully transform health care delivery, hospital leaders must be aware of payment incentives for other providers. In particular, how payment incentives for other providers may not align with hospital incentives, creating barriers to innovation. It is often not the financial incentive to try something different, but rather the financial barrier that prevents groups of providers from aligning with another. Hospital utilization measures, and some hospital "quality" measures can be affected by payment incentives for other providers.

B. McCone, B.A., M.H.A. (✉)
Department of Rate Setting, Maryland Hospital Association,
6820 Deerpath Road, Elkridge, MD 21075, USA
e-mail: bmccone@mhaonline.org

© Springer International Publishing Switzerland 2017   7
H.C. Sax (ed.), *Measurement and Analysis in Transforming Healthcare
Delivery*, DOI 10.1007/978-3-319-46222-6_2

At their core, hospital performance measures provide clinical, financial, and operational leaders tools to manage the daily hospital business, and tools to improve the long-term efficiency and effectiveness of health care delivery. Clear, accurate, and timely data capture is essential to any performance measure. Data building blocks for hospital measurement include basic cost accounting, to complex documentation and coding. In all cases, the measures are subject to the validity of the data reported, requiring examination of a measure's use to address variation among hospitals, within a specific hospital over time, or both.

Overview

This chapter outlines performance measures in *three categories: financial measures, clinical measures, and "combination" measures that attempt to address hospital value.* By definition, the first two categories are easily segregated. The last category may reflect volume, service mix, service use, or a combination of any of these, plus measures that are part clinical and part financial. Additionally, performance measure uses are discussed. Use of the measure may dictate the best application, e.g., absolute performance of hospitals relative to one another, or individual hospital performance over time. Other considerations include defining hospital "costs" as hospital expenditures, versus hospital payments, or costs to health plans and other payers for services rendered.

On the surface, hospital financial measures are straightforward calculations involving easily reportable data. Basic unit cost measures have been used by hospitals for years to manage operations, from supply spending to departmental efficiency. However, unit costs, or prices paid for hospital expenditures, reflect only one driver of hospital costs. The other driver of hospital costs is the volume of services used. Beginning with resource use under a per admission payment system, and ending with resource use in a per capita model, the volume of services used can have a profound effect on hospital costs and hospital payments.

Cost measures only make up the denominator in the value equation. *To provide value, hospitals must also demonstrate high quality.* Clinical performance measures are used to evaluate the quality of hospital care provided during the stay. These measures are generally classified into either *process measures—did you do something* evidence based to improve the patient's health, or *outcome measures—did the patient get better or worse* as a result of the hospital stay. In both categories, the underlying data inputs are crucial to how the measures are viewed and how they change over time.

"Combination" measures may encompass a wide range of calculations to determine relative performance. A simple utilization measure used to compare hospitals is case-mix adjusted length of stay, designed to measure hospital inpatient efficiency while adjusting for differences in service mix. On a case mix adjusted length of stay basis, the hospital will look more efficient with a decline in patient days. At a broader level, the same hospital may look no more or less efficient on a case mix adjusted admission basis if variable costs, or payment levels, do not decline with the decline in patient days. In a payment system with strong financial incentives to reduce readmissions, a measure of clinical effectiveness, the hospital may actually keep the patient the same or even longer, if doing so avoids a readmission. In this case, the marginal cost of keeping the patient an extra day must be lower than the financial penalty of having the patient return to the hospital for a second admission.

Payment incentives to hospitals, and, payment incentives to other providers, affect the overall cost of care. In the example above, the hospital may reduce length of stay to improve inpatient efficiency by simply shifting service use to another setting like skilled nursing care or home health. The hospital generates a cost savings but there is a cost increase with the other service use. Depending on the downstream provider's financial incentives, the other provider's cost of care may be below, the same, or above the truncated hospital use. In the readmission example, the hospital faces two different financial incentives from Medicare. The hospital will receive payment for the additional admission (provided it is not a hospital acquired condition) yet could be subject to a penalty from Medicare if overall readmissions at the hospital place it in the bottom quartile of national readmission rates.

Finally, *the underlying data captured to report hospital performance measures is an important, if not the most important, driver of results.* Hospital financial data tend to be system generated and then analyzed on a per unit, per day, or per admission basis. These cost data are derived from the hospital's underlying direct and indirect cost. The direct cost of supplies and other items is easily tracked. Allocating hospital overhead to calculate unit costs including indirect costs is subject to the method of allocation. Clinical measures tend to come from hospital abstract data and are manually reported, e.g., Medicare value-based purchasing data, or from hospital medical record data that rely on physician documentation and the efficacy of hospital coding. Both areas deserve scrutiny to determine real effect on performance measures as they involve manual data capture and a level of professional judgment from the physician and the coder. Data used for risk-adjusted hospital comparisons is subject to availability and consistency across hospital, state, and national sources.

Financial Measures

Hospital financial measures have long been used to assess hospital performance, for both individual departments and the overall hospital. Hospitals with effective cost accounting systems can accurately track changes in unit cost performance over time. On an aggregate basis, hospitals can compare the cost of an admission or adjusted admission to each other, usually with some risk adjustment. However, the underlying cost per unit measures may be vastly different without the same cost allocations. At a very high level, one can also compare hospital and health care costs on a per beneficiary or per capita basis, though there are a number of factors that influence the validity of the denominator in this measure.

Table 2.1 Unit cost and direct cost

	Unit of Measure	Direct cost per unit	Units	Total cost
Med/surg unit	Patient days	$800.00	3	$2,400
Radiology	RVU's	20.00	50	1,000
Operating room	Minutes	40.00	75	3,000
Anesthesia	Minutes	0.50	75	38
Supplies	Direct Cost	15,000.00	1	15,000
Drugs	Direct Cost	100.00	1	100
Total cost per admission				$21,538

Unit Cost Measurement

At a basic level, hospitals can calculate the per unit input cost of service delivery. Table 2.1 provides an illustration of the direct cost per unit involved in an inpatient stay.

Even this is an inexact science since the staffing costs are typically averaged by dividing nursing unit expenses by the overall volume for a given period. The same is true for ancillary service use, though relative value units (RVUs) are used to equate the intensity of the service performed. Medical supply and drug costs can be calculated based on the actual use of billable supplies. Non-chargeable supplies, while usually 100 % variable, are likely lumped into billable supply costs, charged to the nursing unit and spread over the number of patients served.

Table 2.1 reflects the estimated direct cost of a total joint replacement. As shown in Table 2.1, the hospital incurred $21,538 amount for the overall stay. Of this amount, $15,000 was consumed in direct supply cost. The other direct costs for nursing and ancillary personnel are semi-variable as some level of minimum staffing is required to keep the unit open.[1] From a performance measurement standpoint, the hospital can compute the input costs per unit and try to improve its unit cost efficiency by reducing the input cost of supplies, labor, or both. While it may be difficult to compare absolute cost performance at this level to other hospitals, the hospital can easily measure its cost performance over time to determine if certain initiatives are working.

Table 2.2 reflects the results of two recent programs implemented by the hospital.

First, the hospital implemented a different staffing mix, increasing the number of nurse extenders and decreasing the number of nurses. This resulted in an average savings of $100 per day, or a 13 % reduction in direct room and board costs. Second, the hospital implemented a standardized supply program, reducing the cost of the implant used by $3,000, or 20 %. Overall all, the direct cost for the patient was reduced by 15 %, largely driven by the reduction in supply cost. Since these compu-

---

[1] For an excellent explanation of direct and indirect costs, and, fixed, variable, and semi-variable costs in hospitals, see Health Care Budgeting and Financial Management, Second Edition William J. Ward, Jr. Praeger, an imprint of ABC-CLIO ISBN 978-1-4408-4428-7.

Table 2.2 Direct cost before and after hospital cost reduction programs

	Before hospital programs			After hospital programs			
	Direct cost per unit	Units	Total cost	Direct cost per unit	Units	Total cost	Savings (%)
Med/surg unit	$800.00	3	$2,400	$700.00	3	$2,100	13
Radiology	20.00	50	1,000	20.00	50	1,000	0
Operating room	40.00	75	3,000	40.00	75	3,000	0
Anesthesia	0.50	75	38	0.50	75	38	0
Supplies	15,000.00	1	15,000	12,000.00	1	12,000	20
Drugs	100.00	1	100	100.00	1	100	0
Total cost per admission			$21,538			$18,238	15
Cost savings						$3,300	

tations reflect only a change in unit costs and not underlying volume, there is no need to adjust for the variability of costs with volume.

Table 2.3 overlays the indirect hospital costs. Indirect costs include pure fixed costs (depreciation, interest) and other highly fixed costs (administration, compliance, malpractice expense).

After adjusting for the indirect cost allocation, the total cost of the original example is now $29,076. When the savings programs are implemented, the hospital cost reduction was the same in absolute dollars, but the percentage savings was lower because the overall cost base is higher.

As reflected in the examples, hospitals can measure the unit cost inputs within the same service, with or without adjusting for indirect cost. Per unit costs are useful when measuring the performance of cost reduction initiatives over time, at particular location. The data are easy to gather and use to compute the result, assuming the same use.

Per Admission Measures

The next aggregation of hospital cost measurement is typically on a per admission basis. Unlike the unit cost example, the per admission measure has two cost input variables—unit cost and the number of units of service used during the stay. When aggregating data from multiple patients within a single service line, the data may also be risk or service mix adjusted, based on Medicare Severity Diagnosis Related Groups (MSDRGs) or some other equivalent of service mix.[2] More importantly, if the payment is the same on a per admission basis regardless of the utilization, any reduction in utilization should produce a financial return.

---

[2] The term "case mix" is also used interchangeably, referencing an admission or "case" admitted to the hospital.

Table 2.3 Direct and indirect costs before and after hospital cost reduction programs

	Before hospital programs				After hospital programs				
	Direct cost per unit	Indirect cost per unit	Units	Total cost	Direct cost per unit	Indirect cost per unit	Units	Total cost	Savings (%)
Med/surg unit	$800.00	$280.00	3	$3,240	$700.00	$280.00	3	$2,940	9
Radiology	20.00	7.00	50	1,350	20.00	7.00	50	1,350	0
Operating room	40.00	14.00	75	4,050	40.00	14.00	75	4,050	0
Anesthesia	0.50	0.18	75	51	0.50	0.18	75	51	0
Supplies	15,000.00	5250.00	1	20,250	12,000.00	5,250.00	1	17,250	15
Drugs	100.00	35.00	1	135	100.00	35.00	1	135	0
Total cost per admission					$29,076			$25,776	11
Cost savings								$3,300	

Table 2.4 reflects the same example used in the unit cost analysis.

In this case, the hospital recently improved its discharge efficiency and reduced its length of stay from 3 days to 2 days. However, we also introduce cost variability into the equation. As underlying volume increases or decreases, percentages of the direct and indirect costs are fixed, remaining constant with the change in volume. For illustrative purposes, we will assume that 80 % of the nursing costs are variable, reflecting some portion of fixed staffing cost on the nursing unit. In real world management, nursing unit costs reflect a "step function." In a step function, costs are fixed until the increase or decrease in volume justifies opening or closing of a nursing unit, respectively. We also assume that 90 % of the indirect overhead costs, administration, patient accounting, etc., are fixed as they remain relatively unchanged with volume. In this example, the other costs are fixed as they are assumed to be provided on the first or second day (surgery, X-ray, etc.).

As shown in Table 2.4, the hospital generated a 2 % cost reduction per admission by reducing the length of stay from 3 days to 2 days. On an individual admission, the financial performance improved slightly when compared to the unit cost example. If length-of-stay improvements are generated on a wide basis, the cost effect multiplies, particularly if declining volumes result in closing a unit as reflected in the step function. Some of the indirect cost is also further reduced (e.g., dietary, housekeeping, etc.), compounding the savings. As an alternative to closing a unit, additional financial benefits may accrue if the now empty beds are back filled with patients waiting in the queue for services.

The per admission measure can be useful when comparing costs among physicians in the hospital or when comparing costs across hospitals. Using Medicare case mix index (CMI), the hospital can aggregate patients by physician in a particular service line as a useful tool to compare the average cost per patient.[3] Comparing aggregate hospital efficiency can be accomplished by aggregating expenses generally (all hospital expenses per discharge) or by aggregating expenses for a particular service if the data are available (e.g., orthopedics, total joint replacements, etc.).

Table 2.5 compares case mix adjusted cost per admission between two physicians, assumed to practice the same type of service (orthopedics) but with a different mix of cases. Assume the two physicians perform only two types of cases, total joint

---

[3] Though CMI is a measure of the severity of cases treated, it is not a perfect measure. Medicare CMI is a measure of average resource use, based on the grouping of admissions into categories with similar service use (e.g., total joint replacement, influenza, etc.). However, the underlying case weights assigned to a particular MSDRG are based on Medicare claims data and therefore reflect Medicare patients only. Discharges from other payers may reflect higher or lower resource use. Applying Medicare CMI to compare all payer per admission costs across hospitals may not accurately reflect the true service mix as the patient populations can vary. MSDRGs though severity adjusted, measure severity adjusted resource use as determined by Medicare payments, and may not reflect patient complexity if applied to all patients. Other groupers, such as the 3M's All Patient Refined Diagnostic Related Group (APRDRG) logic use different coding logic and different groupings. Case weights may also vary depending on the discharges used to predict the underlying resource use. State Medicaid programs use different grouping logics and a different patient population than the Medicare grouper.

Table 2.4 Direct and Indirect Costs, Volume Changes, and Volume Variability

	Before hospital programs						After hospital programs						
	Direct cost per unit	% Variable	Indirect cost per unit	% Variable	Units	Total cost	Direct cost per unit	% Variable	Indirect cost per unit	% Variable	Units	Total cost	Savings (%)
Med/surg unit	$800.00	80	$280.00	10	3	$3240	$800.00	80	$280.00	10	2	$2572	21
Radiology	20.00	80	7.00	10	50	1350	20.00	80	7.00	10	50	1,350	0
Operating room	40.00	80	14.00	10	75	4050	40.00	80	14.00	10	75	4,050	0
Anesthesia	0.50	90	0.18	10	75	51	0.50	90	0.18	10	75	51	0
Supplies	15,000.00	95	5,250.00	10	1	20,250	15,000.00	95	5,250.00	10	1	20,250	0
Drugs	100.00	95	35.00	10	1	135	100.00	95	35.00	10	1	135	0
Total cost per admission						$29,076						$28,408	2
Cost savings												$668	

Table 2.5 Case mix adjusted cost per admission

	Physician 1	Physician 2
Average length of stay	5	3
Total costs	$750,000	$500,000
Total admissions	10	10
Unadjusted cost per admission	$75,000	$50,000
Medicare CMI	5.00	3.00
Case mix adjusted cost per admission	$15,000	$16,667

replacements (lower intensity) and spinal reconstruction (higher intensity). Using these assumptions, we can measure efficiency on a relative, per admission basis.

In this comparison, Physician 1 admitted 10 patients with an average length of stay of 5 days, with total costs of $750,000, or $75,000 per admission. Physician 2 also admitted 10 patients with an average length of stay of 3 days, with total costs of $500,000, or $50,000 per admission. Physician 1 reflected a case mix of 5.0, for a case mix adjusted cost per admission of $15,000. Physician 2 reflected a case mix of 3.0, for a case mix adjusted cost per admission of $16,667. On an unadjusted basis, Physician 1's cost per case is 50 % higher than Physician 2's cost per case. After adjusting for CMI, Physician 1's cost per case is actually 10 % lower than Physician 2's cost per case. *A strong understanding of risk adjustment is vital in evaluation of individual physicians as well as negotiating prospective payments.*

Per Capita or per Beneficiary Measures

At the highest level, hospital costs can be measured on a per beneficiary or a per capita basis. This type of measure is best used to compare aggregate costs for a group of hospitals in a wide geographic area. For example, statewide total hospital cost or the statewide total hospital payments could be calculated, divided by the total population, resulting in a per capita cost/payment that could be compared to other states. (Note: in-migration and out-migration will affect the denominator). The same measure could also be used to determine per beneficiary costs or payments for a defined number of beneficiaries in a health plan.

Unlike unit costs or even per admission costs, per capita spending is much more likely to be affected by the use of services rather than the underlying service cost. The Medicare Accountable Care Organization (ACO) model seeks to align incentives by improving population health and reducing avoidable resource use, rewarding the ACO with financial incentives that can be shared with the participating providers. The new Maryland All-Payer model uses the same concept to measure hospital spending, both on a per capita basis and on a Medicare per beneficiary basis.

Table 2.6 compares the year-over-year hospital spending performance of State A on a per capita basis. In this example, State A reduced hospital spending by reducing

Table 2.6 Year over year statewide hospital spending per discharge and statewide hospital spending per capita

State A	Year 1	Year 2	Change	% Change
Hospital payments	$10,000,000,000	$9,660,000,000	$(340,000,000)	−3.4
Discharges	800,000	736,000	(64,000)	−8.0
Payment per discharge	$12,500	$13,125	$625	5.0
Hospital payments	$10,000,000,000	$9,660,000,000	$(340,000,000)	−3.4
Population	5,900,000	6,077,000	177,000	3.0
Payment per capita	$1,695	$1,590	$(105)	−6.2

hospital discharges by 8% while per admission costs actually rose. (For illustrative purposes, this assumes net zero in-migration and out-migration for hospital services.)

This type of measure is a departure from the historic focus on unit cost and per admission utilization controls. It is consistent with the triple aim goal to reduce costs by reducing per capita spending [2], regardless of the underlying cost inputs. The data may or may not be case mix adjusted, depending on the use. The Maryland model does not adjust for service mix. Rather it sets a fixed, annual growth ceiling for all payer per capita spending, and a variable Medicare per beneficiary spending target, relative to national hospital spending per beneficiary growth.

The Maryland demonstration model is in its third year. Though early in its implementation, the model has demonstrated early progress by exceeding the required targets in year 1 [3]. As service delivery evolves under this model, one might expect consolidation of services, particularly at hospitals with lower volumes that result in higher fixed costs. In other single payer countries, complex procedures are often cohorted at fewer locations to allocate indirect and fixed costs over a larger volume base. The impact of the new Maryland model on the hospital delivery is underway, though it may be several years before these significant types of market movements occur.

Hospital Clinical Quality Measures

As the US health care system transforms from volume to value, clinical performance measures play an increasingly important role in hospital management, payment incentive design and consumer awareness. Clinical performance measures tend to fall into two categories: evidence-based process of care (process) measures and outcome measures, though there is not a strict definition. A third category, patient perception of the hospital stay is by definition an "outcome measure," reflecting how the patient *felt* about his or her stay in the hospital. However, these are not clinical outcomes—hospital acquired infection, mortality, etc. There are advantages and disadvantages to either category, depending on the context of measure use. Both clinical measure categories begin with the same idea: how do we quantify "hospital quality" to inform hospital stakeholders. *Over time, the focus on hospital performance has migrated to outcome measures, but there is conflicting evidence that measuring outcomes alone can improve quality* [4].

One challenge of using clinical performance measures is the sheer volume of quality data collected. QualityNet.org identifies and organizes CMS quality measures for different types of service providers [5]. Though comprehensive for CMS, other payers may require different data reporting. Hospital resources are consumed because of the vast reporting required. Hospital resources are not only used to collect and report quality data, but also to review, validate, audit, secure, and most importantly leverage the data to improve the hospital's relative performance.

This section focuses on CMS's Acute Care Hospital Quality Improvement Program Measures since they are consistent across all US hospitals. There are four main CMS quality incentive programs in the CMS quality improvement environment. They include:

- Hospital Inpatient Quality Reporting (IQR) program
- Hospital Value-Based Purchasing (VBP)
- Hospital-Acquired Condition Reduction Program (HACRP)
- Hospital Readmissions Reduction Program (HRRP)

These four programs combine both process and outcome measures. In addition to these programs, clinical performance measures are released on CMS's HospitalCompare website for public consumption.

Process Measures

Process of care measures emerged as the first generation of clinical data used to measure hospital performance. Medicare's Inpatient Quality Reporting (IQR) program was implemented in 2003 as part of the Prescription Drug Act. Initially, hospitals were required to submit process of care data to Medicare or receive a 0.4% reduction to the annual Medicare Inpatient Prospective Payment System (IPPS) payment update. In 2008, hospitals faced a 2.0% reduction to the annual payment update if the data were not reported.

Process measures used by CMS have evolved over time, based on the effectiveness of their adoption. A current IQR process measure is Fibrinolytic Therapy Received Within 30 min of Hospital Arrival for acute myocardial infarction (AMI) patients. Fibrinolytic therapy is a proven treatment for the management of AMI, reflecting improved outcomes by following the process [6]. Prior to 2015, there were several process measures for AMI treatment originally in IQR, including Aspirin at arrival and Beta-Blocker prescribed at discharge. These measures have been removed, not because they were determined to be ineffective, but because they were "topped out," as being followed close to 100% of the time by all hospitals. These process measures are now voluntarily reported.

As referenced in the fibrinolytic therapy example, process of care measures are clinically accepted based on published and peer reviewed evidence. Once determined to be effective, the treatment protocol can be built into a hospital's process of care, with the expectation that the process will improve patient outcomes. As hospitals continually move toward value-based care delivery, process measures should be constantly plotted with respect to outcomes, to validate that the supposed process improvements are improving health outcomes. The topped out measures suggest that hospitals are following accepted process measures, yet outcomes could vary, reflecting other clinical improvements or different patient populations that appear similar on the surface.

Outcome Measures

One definition of a health care outcome measure states it as a measure of quality of medical care, the standard against which the end result of the intervention is assessed [7]. Another non-health care source defines an outcome measure as the determination and evaluation of the results of an activity, plan, process, or program and their comparison with the intended or projected results [8]. In either case, the outcome can be defined as the *result* of something.

Hospital outcome measures may apply to different patient populations within the hospital. Certain outcome measures have a limited denominator, or patient pool from which the measure is applied. For example, CMS is collecting hospital 30-day, all-cause mortality rates following AMI hospitalizations. In this example, the pool of patients is limited to patients that were hospitalized for AMI. Expanding further, CMS measures rates for central line-associated bloodstream infections (CLABSI) and catheter-associated urinary tract infections (CAUTI). These outcome measures reflect the entire pool of patients at the hospital, minus those admitted with an infection.

It is critical to understand how outcome measures can be affected by hospital interventions, the nature of the population and the intersection of both. One process measure is use of prophylactic antibiotics received within 1 h prior to surgical incision, a clinical or hospital intervention. It can be assumed that following this intervention should lead to better performance on various outcome measures including surgical site infections, or in the near term, hospital readmission for surgical site infections. Other outcome measures, such as 30-day readmission rate for heart failure patients may correlate with the severity of the patient population. Even of all process of care measures are followed during the initial hospital stay, if the patient has significant underlying complications, the readmission rate may be higher. Case mix adjustments can be used to risk adjust the population used in the 30-day heart failure readmission example, but CMI may not fully adjust for all underlying clinical differences.

Defining Value: The Intersection of Financial and Quality Measures

After separately exploring both financial and quality measures, we turn to applying both to determine hospital value. Value may be determined in the aggregate, overall cost versus overall quality, or in subcategories, process measures followed versus resulting outcomes. In both cases, the goal is to determine value, or the quality of care for the cost, or payment, incurred.

At the highest level, a simple way to examine value is to use an *XY* plot of hospital cost versus outcomes. Figure 2.1 reflects an aggregate plot of hospital cost per admission versus a composite outcome score.

In this example, there are four quadrants, relative to the average of the hospitals measured: high cost/high quality, high cost/low quality, low cost/high quality, and low cost/low quality. Though crude, this measure provides basic illustration of value.

On the cost side, a hospital's cost or payment per admission is inherently weighted by the average of all costs or payments for the patient population. Therefore, a hospital with a higher proportion of normal deliveries relative to intensive surgical procedures is expected to have a lower overall cost per admission. Developing a composite outcome measure is more subjective, depending on the method of weighting each outcome. Weighting the outcomes equally is one method, while a different method might weight the outcomes on the volume of each patient pool reflected in the outcome. In the normal delivery versus surgical case example, if the hospital has a higher proportion of deliveries, then one might weight the percentage of obstetric patients higher to weight the percentage of obstetric complications higher.

Adjusting one or both sides of the measures (cost or quality) may reveal a different picture. For example, large academic medical centers typically have higher

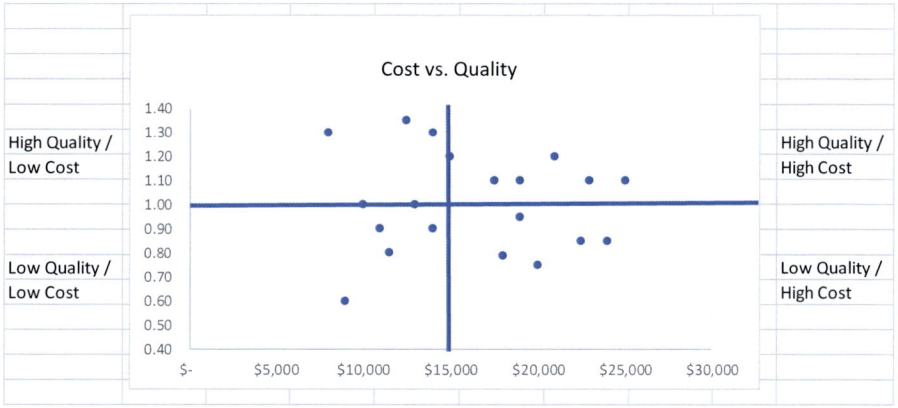

Fig. 2.1 Cost versus quality

costs than smaller community hospitals for three reasons: mix of patients, teaching costs, and disproportionate share costs. The first reason is straightforward, as academic medical centers tend to treat the most difficult and complex patients. The other two reasons affect cost both directly—actual resident salary costs, and indirectly—the underlying utilization from clinical training and from treating a poor population. As an example, the aggregate hospital cost measure could be adjusted by the percentage of Medicare add on payments for IME and DSH, attempting to eliminate the variation.

When adjusting the value measure, it is important to understand the actual measures used in the plot. Many clinical outcome measures are inherently risk or case mix adjusted, eliminating the need to further adjust for service mix differences. On the cost side, it could be argued that costs should also be adjusted by service mix to reflect the resources used to treat the hospital's patients. Depending of the use of the value measure, both may be valid. The unadjusted measure may be used to strictly determine quality as a result of spending, while the adjusted measure may be used to justify variation in costs related to underlying circumstances, e.g., the social benefits from additional resource use, such as physician training or treating an underprivileged population.

Below the aggregate level, the value measure can be divided into subclassifications related to hospital specialties. For example, a hospital specializing in open heart procedures may want to analyze its value relative to other open heart hospitals by comparing the average cost per discharge for AMI patients versus the 30-day readmission rate. In this example, the comparison attempts to limit the value proposition to a single specialty reflected in the purpose of the comparison.

If the cost and quality variables are analyzed separately, it may not be a value measure by simple definition, but could still prove instructive. For example, one could analyze the process of care measures versus outcomes to focus on the clinical quality. Plotting fibrinolytic therapy versus 30-day AMI readmissions is an example of this. On the cost side, one could analyze case mix adjusted length of stay versus the overall cost per admission to determine if length of stay is a predictor of costs. Over time, if length of stay decreases, one would expect the overall cost per case mix adjusted admission to decrease.

Payment Incentives and Underlying Data

Payment Incentives

When using hospital performance measures, payment incentives, whether for hospitals or for other providers, can impact cost and quality. Medicare's IPPS is based on an average payment per admission. Therefore, if a hospital reduces length of stay or other underlying resource use and in theory, the associated variable costs, the hospital becomes more efficient by retaining a higher marginal return on each per discharge payment. The hospital, especially if part of a larger integrated delivery system, may use other services such as skilled nursing or home health to discharge patients to a lower cost setting, improving the hospital's performance.

In this example, one should examine the downstream financial and quality outcomes. On the quality side, analyzing the patient population in cohorts may be instructive to the resulting outcomes. For example, break the hospital discharges into several categories: discharges to skilled nursing, discharges to home health, and discharges to home. Plotting the hospital readmission rate from each classification may help the hospital identify areas of focus, if the readmissions rate from one classification is higher than the others. As discussed previously, a service mix adjustment from the pool of discharges might be applied to normalize for the variation in patient populations discharged to the various services.

In another example, length of stay could be plotted against the hospital's readmission rate in the aggregate or for a particular specialty. If the readmission payment incentive is stronger than the per admission efficiency incentive, the hospital might analyze length of stay to determine if keeping the patient longer is actually *more* efficient than improving hospital service use. If the readmission rate declines with longer length of stay, it would suggest that the additional length of stay is beneficial to reducing readmissions. Though they are both considered to be hospital performance measures, the two payment incentives must be thoroughly analyzed to determine the most efficient service use.

Another downstream effect may be to compare hospital spending to total spending, understanding the divergent nature of payment incentives. For example, if the hospital reduces length of stay by discharging patients to a skilled nursing provider near the end of the hospital stay, the hospital may improve its efficiency. However, if the skilled nursing provider is paid on a per diem basis, it does not have the same incentive as the hospital to reduce its length of stay. Medicare payments to SNFs are based on resource use per day, with a certain limit. Even with resource adjustments, the SNF is paid on a per day basis, in theory, with a financial incentive to keep the patient until the benefit expires. Here, the hospital may reduce length of stay by a few days, but it might lead to a longer stay in SNF than the last few days of the hospital stay.

On a per capita or per beneficiary spending basis, differing payment incentives may affect the total spending per capital or per beneficiary. Maryland's All-Payer model requires that the state generate $330 million in hospital savings over 5 years by maintaining the growth in hospital spending per Maryland Medicare beneficiary below the national average. Additionally, Maryland hospitals are limited to an annual global budget, or a fixed hospital revenue amount per year, no matter the change in hospital use. However, the All-Payer model also limits the growth in total spending per Maryland beneficiary to the growth in national spending per Medicare beneficiary over 2 years. Thus, Maryland hospitals are incentivized to reduce hospital use, but the Medicare total spending guardrail means that replacing hospital use with other services must result in overall system efficiency, not just hospital efficiency. CMS is also evaluating this type of total cost of care guardrail in other models, such as hospital physician gainsharing arrangements.

Underlying Data

Though the focus of this chapter is on the application and use of hospital performance measures, the underlying data used in these measures is critical to reflect
actual performance. Without the appropriate data capture and reporting, hospital
performance on a given measure may vary from period to period.

The data used for hospital measures are generally garnered from five sources:

- Medical records
- Patient surveys
- Hospital claims
- Hospital surveys
- Hospital costs

These five sources result in the data captured and reported on a variety of clinical
and financial measures.

Medical records and hospital claims are used to determine performance on most
clinical quality measures. Relying on documentation and coding, the medical record
is the primary source used for underlying process of care and clinical outcome measures or a per patient basis. *The importance of timely, accurate physician, and nursing documentation cannot be overstated for its effect on performance measures.* In
particular, conditions present on admission must be captured and reported.
Otherwise the hospital's scores for hospital acquired conditions may be inaccurate.
Medical record data abstraction involves manually capturing data from the medical
record for reporting on process of care measures, whether the data are input into an
electronic database such as Medicare's Electronic Clinical Quality Measurement
(eCQM) format or reported separately. Abstracting personnel require appropriate
training and oversight, and the hospital should review or audit the abstractions for
accuracy.

Hospital claims data are used to measure aggregate patient outcomes and may
also be used to aggregate payments to measure payment per unit of service. These
data are generally more straightforward and easier to capture than medical record
data, but are still critically important. Clinical performance measures such as 30-day
measures of mortality and hospital readmissions are derived from claims data.
Payment levels captured reflect third-party payment for services and may be aggregated on measures of financial performance. If both cases, accurate medical record
numbers, dates of service, and charging will affect the resulting measures.

Patient surveys and hospital surveys are used to capture Hospital Consumer
Assessment of Healthcare Providers and Systems (HCAHPS) and National Health
Safety Network (NHSN) data. HCAHPS data reflect the patient's view of their treatment in the hospital, and may be more subjective because these data are based on a
patient's perception of their hospital treatment. The NHSN survey data are used in
structural measures of hospital effectiveness, such as the Hospital Survey on Patient
Safety Culture and the Safe Surgery Checklist. Hospitals should have adequate processes in place to collect and report these data on a timely and accurate basis.

Hospital cost data are typically generated by hospital financial and information systems to capture the expenses of patient care. As outlined in the cost measures section, costs can be measured on a per unit, a per admission, or an overall hospital basis. The level of sophistication of any hospital's cost accounting, decision support, or other systems vary, making it difficult to compare performance across hospitals. Since the inception of cost-based reimbursement dating back to the late 1960s and early 1970s, the annual Medicare cost report summarizes the direct patient care and indirect overhead costs by hospital. Hospitals can use these data for cost comparison purposes, since it is relatively prescriptive for cost allocation. These data are aggregated in CMS's Hospital Cost Report Information System (HCRIS) data, summarized by Medicare cost center.

Conclusion

There are endless ways to define and measure hospital performance. Both cost and clinical quality measures serve as the basic inputs to the value equation. Hospital leaders, regulators, health plans, and other stakeholders should understand the use and application of the measure in question, along with understanding the payment incentives and data that drive performance.

References

1. Porter ME. What is value in health care? N Engl J Med. 2010;363:2477–8.
2. Berwick DM, Nolan TW, Whittington J. The triple aim: care, health, and cost. Health Aff. 2008;27(3):759–69.
3. Ankit P, Rajkumar R, Colmers JM, Kinzer D, Conway PH, Sharfstein J. Maryland's global hospital budgets—preliminary results from an all-payer mode. N Engl J Med. 2015;373:20.
4. Burton T. Why process measures are often more important than outcome measures in healthcare. Health Catalyst. Presentation, December 8, 2014.
5. https://www.qualitynet.org/dcs/ContentServer?c=Page&pagename=QnetPublic%2FPage%2F QnetTier3&cid=1138900297065
6. Rivera-Bou WL, Brown DFM. Thrombolytic therapy. Medscape; 2014.
7. Mosby's medical dictionary, 9th ed. St. Louis: Elsevier; 2009.
8. http://www.businessdictionary.com/definition/outcome-measure.html

Chapter 3
Measurements and Analysis in Transforming Healthcare Delivery: Terminology and Applications—Physician Performance

David Norris

Introduction

Performance is defined as the execution of a plan. For physicians, that plan is to keep or make patients healthy. How well physicians do this is described as "physician performance."

It is important to appreciate this fundamental definition of physician performance because it has—up until recently—been poorly understood. Internal data held by hospitals have not been shared publicly. Therefore in the past, performance measures were delineated with a 1–5-star consumer review, much the way a restaurant is reviewed. But this rating system is subjective and seriously flawed. It can include everything from the availability of parking to the attitude of the office staff. It does not offer a meaningful view of a physician's actual performance and it limits a patient's ability to evaluate their physician choices.

Government agencies are now requiring a more complete picture of physician performance, and consumers are seeking a more empowering tool for choosing their doctors. These demands are giving rise to physician performance transparency, an effective and useful means to evaluate the quality of a physician's work.

New technology is available to factually represent the historical performance of physicians—their experience, outcomes, and efficiency. The intelligent analysis of big data is, for the first time, giving consumers and health systems valuable new tools in rating and selecting healthcare providers.

Impartial, data-driven performance evaluations were once exclusively reserved for hospitals and health systems. From Leapfrog to the Joint Commission, organizations and mechanisms abound to determine the quality and effectiveness of a hospital. But within every medical center are physicians charged with delivering quality care.

D. Norris, B.S.-C.S. (✉)
MD Insider, 3015 Main st., Suite 333, Santa Monica, CA 90405, USA
e-mail: david.norris.x@gmail.com

© Springer International Publishing Switzerland 2017
H.C. Sax (ed.), *Measurement and Analysis in Transforming Healthcare Delivery*, DOI 10.1007/978-3-319-46222-6_3

It is the physician who must make the right call in an emergency, the surgeon who must master their skills and the oncologist who must make the correct diagnosis in order for care to be deemed "good."

Data surrounding physician performance are finally reflecting that reality. It is aligning the industry understanding of quality with the way patients have always understood it: at the individual physician level.

Rather than solely focusing on institutional outcomes, consumers—along with the Centers for Medicare & Medicaid Services—are turning the spotlight on physician outcomes, and on comparing the fundamental differences between the expertise and experience of physicians who perform the same types of procedures.

At the end of 2015, CMS published its Quality Measure Development Plan, a framework to develop clinician quality measurements, which it touted as exemplifying the shift in Medicare payments "from volume to value" [1].

CMS plans to use these data to support a Merit-Based Incentive Payment System (MIPS), which will calculate Medicare payment adjustments on a composite performance score across four categories, including the quality of care. How well a doctor does his or her job seems like an obvious category to include in an incentive program, but until the advent of electronic medical records, quantifying quality was impossible. Now, it is a matter of ones and zeroes.

The result of all these performance data will be a better-informed consumer population that can make fact-based decisions about their healthcare. It will lead to lowered error rates, fewer readmissions, and lower healthcare costs. And it will likely inject a healthy dose of competition between providers, one that elevates the performance of all physicians.

The source of physician performance data is at once elegant and enormous. Billions of rows of claims data generated commercially are now available for anyone to see. Of course, sifting through dizzying amounts of data is not exactly easy and models for creating meaningful analysis of performance have come under scrutiny. Government models, in particular, are criticized for inaccuracies and misleading information. But other models exist that generate verifiable data reflective of the true level of physician performance quality.

Data scientists have developed industry-vetted algorithms that provide intelligent, *risk-adjusted* ratings of physician performance. These ratings are based on experience, outcomes, comorbidities, risk factors, caseloads, and a myriad of other factors. Complications, readmissions, length of stay, and patient experiences are also taken into account to provide a comprehensive view into the performance of nearly every physician in the country—giving patients and health systems the details they need to make informed decisions about healthcare providers.

Even before the Affordable Care Act, the healthcare industry has been interested in unlocking this information. Patients can learn nearly everything about the diseases that ail them, but nearly nothing about the physicians who treat them. Health systems are at the mercy of providers who either follow the standard of care or who do not. A surgeon's website can list awards, affiliations, and years out of medical school, but there is nothing in their CV that indicates whether they have great outcomes or not. Physician performance provides those critical details—the information that separates reputation from fact, and can mean the difference between life and death.

That is why understanding physician performance represents one of the most significant changes in healthcare—and one of the most important aspects of the healthcare overhaul.

What Is the Need for Performance Information?

To encourage performance transparency, we must first gather performance information. Government agencies have been working for years to collect as much data as possible, and commercial ventures, journalists, and advocacy groups have been clamoring for all the information they can gather.

The momentum toward collecting and publicizing performance information will only grow more powerful, as it should. Performance transparency improves outcomes, lowers costs, and enables consumers to make informed decisions [2]. Health systems that stay ahead of this movement will help decide the direction of this trend—and will benefit enormously from the improvements it yields.

For several years, the healthcare industry has been moving away from the fee-for-service model and toward accountable care and value-based pricing. In fact, the American Hospital Association reports that the majority of patients will be part of a risk-based contract, including initiatives such as bundled payments, by 2020 [3]. This will drive narrow networks to align with the highest-quality providers. And it places a greater emphasis on care that is thoughtful, efficient, and cost-effective.

Finding appropriate, high-value care will prove increasingly important. In its case study about the effectiveness of the transition to Accountable Care Organizations, the AHA reported, "Case study leaders unanimously agree that access to all clinical and claims data across the care continuum for their patient population was critical to success" [4].

In other words, without access to intelligent analysis of performance information, health systems cannot move their organizations toward higher quality and lower costs.

Physicians also benefit enormously from the analysis of performance information. The culture of medicine has historically put the physician in charge. They, after all, are the persons who have to lean on their substantial education and experience to make judgment calls about a patient's health. But not all doctors are created equal.

Evidence-based medicine is constantly changing the status quo, rendering obsolete the practices and procedures a physician learned in medical school or during residency. Those physicians who keep up with the evolving standard of care are more likely to benefit from innovation than those providers who are reticent to alter their clinical behaviors.

But change for the sake of change helps no one. Just as physicians need hard data proving the effectiveness of a drug or a procedure before trying it on patients, so will they require substantial data science to convince them of the benefits of performance transparency. Sound data proving transparency's role in reducing adverse outcomes are incredibly compelling and hard to refute.

It will also be critical that performance information solely be used to improve the standard of care—not to embarrass or punish individual doctors. It should be presented as practice-based aggregated data, and not a contest to judge doctors based on whether they are "good" or "bad."

Researchers at Johns Hopkins in 2015 found that by taking this fact-based, quality-improvement approach, hospitals were able to use real-time feedback and financial incentives to reach higher safety and quality levels in the prevention of venous thromboembolism (VTE) [5].

Physicians took the granular information about their own prevention protocol compliance and risk assessment techniques to identify what they were doing well—and what they needed to improve. The results were fewer cases of VTE developing during hospital stays, and far more compliance with existing protocols. In fact, the percentage of incidents of doctors failing to prescribe proper prevention of VTE dropped from 6.1 to 3.2 % with performance feedback.

While improved care and patient safety are paramount, the catalyst for all these data gathering is the government agencies charged with driving down healthcare costs.

The number most often quoted for representing the annual cost of medical errors is $17.1 billion [6]. In 2008, Medicare released a list of "never events," serious, costly errors in inpatient care that should never happen [7]. These included foreign objects left in the body after surgery, falls and traumas while at a hospital, catheter-associated urinary tract infections; mediastinitis, or inflammation in the area between the lungs, after coronary artery bypass grafting; and pressure ulcers. That same year CMS stopped paying the excess cost for inpatient stays complicated by "never events," but that did not stop the errors from occurring [8]. A 2013 study estimated that more than 4000 surgical "never events" still occur yearly in the United States [8].

Of course the biggest stakeholder in performance transparency is the patient. As consumers of healthcare shoulder more of the cost, patients are becoming savvier and more discerning about the price and quality of their care. They are questioning physicians with greater frequency and "shopping around" more for high-quality physicians who will deliver good outcomes with lower costs and less recovery time.

In 2013 alone, 16.4 % of healthcare spending per individual covered by employer-sponsored insurance was paid out of pocket. *Patients are spending more out-of-pocket on doctor's visits and specialists than ever before* [9]. They also have the most to lose. Every year as many as 440,000 people die in hospitals from preventable errors and poor judgment calls [10]. With the advent of better information gathering, needless deaths and injuries are starting to decline.

In fact, the Agency for Healthcare Research and Quality reported that about 2.1 million fewer patients were harmed in hospitals from infections, adverse drug events and other conditions between 2010 and 2014. The progress on hospital-acquired conditions alone resulted in 87,000 fewer deaths, improvements that the AHRQ largely attributed to a focus on performance information (Fig. 3.1).

Reliance on performance information has resulted in a reduction of some of the most dangerous—and expensive—hospital-acquired conditions.

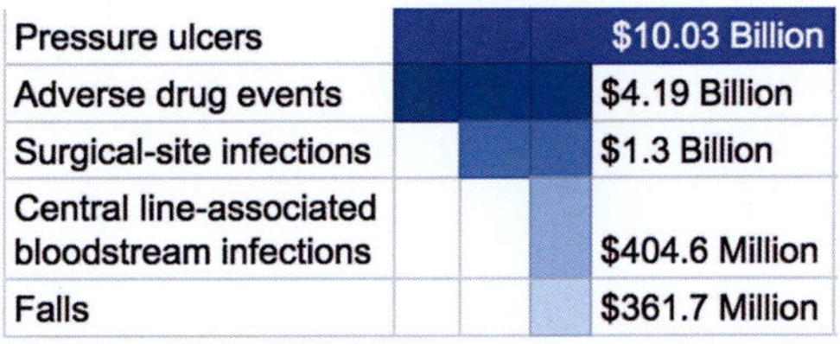

Fig. 3.1 Top five gains on hospital-acquired conditions by costs averted, 2011–2014

Pressure ulcers		$10.03 Billion
Adverse drug events		$4.19 Billion
Surgical-site infections		$1.3 Billion
Central line-associated bloodstream infections		$404.6 Million
Falls		$361.7 Million

Helping patients find the most appropriate physician for them has another, unintended consequence: It improves the patient experience. Instead of wasting time with providers who lack the requisite training, do not have the proper expertise or are just not the right "fit" for a particular patient, patients who are immediately directed to the "best" doctor for them report far better outcomes and report a more satisfying experience.

The New Language of Quality Measurements

We have defined performance, but how do we measure it? As we previously saw, a scientific analysis of performance can help transform the healthcare industry. But because medicine is as much an art as it is a science, physician performance is vulnerable to subjective metrics.

It is imperative, therefore, to understand the existing and emerging quality measurements, their uses, and their limitations.

Quality

What are we talking about when we talk about quality? According to the Institute of Medicine's landmark 1990 report [11], quality is defined as "the degree to which healthcare services for individuals and populations increase the likelihood of desired health outcomes and are consistent with current professional knowledge."

In the 25 years since that report was released, "quality" has also come to mean outcomes, efficiency, value, and preventative health. The role of the physician is changing from treating illness to helping patients avoid getting sick in the first place. In a perspective published in the New England Journal of Medicine, *value* is seen as essentially synonymous with *quality*:

"Achieving high value for patients must become the overarching goal of health-care delivery, with value defined as the health outcomes achieved per dollar spent. This goal is what matters for patients and unites the interests of all actors in the system," writes Michael E. Porter, Ph.D., a Harvard University economist. "There is no substitute for measuring actual outcomes, whose principal purpose is not comparing providers but enabling innovations in care" [12].

Even when "quality" is quantified with data, it can still be subject to bias or misinterpretation. When CMS released its updated Physician Compare data in December 2015 [13], for instance, the American Medical Association criticized it as incomplete and inaccurate because it only accounts for data submitted voluntarily by doctors [13].

For quality measures to truthfully reflect quality of performance, data must be risk-adjusted, standardized, and industry-vetted. It must also take into account experience and patient outcomes, including ancillary procedures and readmission rates.

Transparency

In the early days of reporting, transparency meant raw data. But that is not what consumers need. They need context and comparisons. *Does my doctor have a high mortality rate? Does my doctor have the latest technological advances to treat me in the most effective way possible?* That information then needs to be weighed against similar providers.

Many doctors bristle at the suggestion of comparisons or "grades," but they are unavoidable. Consumer sites as varied as Healthgrades and Yelp provide subjective physician reviews or ratings, based on consumer feedback. These reviews aggregate various aspects of the patient experience, including the pleasantness of the office staff and the number of parking spaces at the doctor's office, giving potential patients information that may or may not be relevant regarding the actual quality of care.

True performance transparency actually helps to counter both the complexity of raw data and the often questionable subjective online reviews. By mining the key information that actually pertains to patient care, physician performance transparency paints a complete picture of a provider's experience, quality, and cost.

(We mention cost because—while most people do not pick a doctor because he or she is the cheapest—cost is a measure that resonates with patients. When combined with expertise, experience, and outcomes, it proves to be an illuminating aspect of performance.)

Currently, outcomes and clinical data information are available from both commercial and CMS sources, but many hospitals are also starting to present their own in-house data for analysis to help improve performance and identify potential cost savings (more on that later). This growth in transparency enhances the sophistication and accuracy of the data, which in turn, leads to more "buy-in" from physicians for increasing transparency.

Patient-Reported Outcomes

While seemingly subjective, patient-reported outcomes help answer the simple question: "Did this doctor make you better?" This is a key quality measurement, and one that often matters most to patients.

Everyone wants to know about the end result. Did the back pain go away? Is the cancer in remission? CMS considers this measure so important, it is requiring long-term care hospitals to survey patients about their outcomes.

If patient satisfaction seems like more of a marketing ploy than an actionable measurement, consider this: An Italian study recently found that breast cancer patients who were given a 10-item questionnaire reported more treatment side effects than their physicians recognized during follow-up examinations—a discrepancy that speaks to the heart of why patient perspectives are so vital [14].

Patient Reported Outcomes (PRO) can help drive institutional changes that directly affect care. For instance, studies have found that patients who are engaged in their care tend to choose less costly but highly effective interventions, such as physical therapy for low back pain.

PROs can even help predict whether patients will be compliant with physician orders. The American Journal of Managed Care reported that at an American College of Cardiology meeting in March 2015 [15], researchers presented promising findings for the drug ticagrelor, used to treat acute coronary syndrome. The researchers noted that the drug reduced the likelihood of heart attacks but might produce "minor bleeding." The scientist dismissed the side effect as inconsequential [15]. But by November, at an American Heart Association meeting, a follow-up presentation found that one-third of the patients in the ticagrelor study stopped taking the drug, despite the fact that it worked [15].

According to AJMC: "Researchers suspect too many found the daily nosebleed insufferable. 'Often in trials we categorize events as non-serious, but they have importance for patients,' said Marc Bonaca, MD, of Brigham and Women's Hospital" [15].

When gathering PROs, it is important to keep innovation—not penalization—in the forefront as the goal. By focusing performance measurement on PROs that are directly related to end results—discomfort, ancillary procedures, quality of life—patient-reported outcomes will help provide an unbiased view of a subjective, but critical, component of physician performance.

After all, patients have the final word on whether an intervention "worked" or did not. Capturing patient perspectives on their own outcomes can help health systems accurately appraise the quality and efficiency of the care patients receive.

Best Practices

Best practices are those policies and procedures that get the right care to the right patient at the right time. By having health systems and physicians identify and implement best practices, government agencies are trying to reduce infections, errors, and preventable bad outcomes. And by following those best practices, the healthcare industry is seeking to standardize quality.

No two patients are exactly alike, so it stands to reason that no two treatment plans will be identical either. However there are gold standards by which it is safe to make blanket judgments: Do physicians wash their hands? Use checklists? Properly scrub down patients before surgery? By paying attention to fundamental best practices, consumers are learning where to go and whom to trust with their care.

"Best" also means "evidenced-based." As medical technology evolves and knowledge advances, it can become difficult to keep track of exactly how well a provider keeps current with the latest evidenced-based medicine. This is where comparisons are particularly helpful: A provider's outcomes relative to her peers can help reveal how up-to-date she is with current advances.

Some of these advances are not even that advanced. In a study published in the *New England Journal of Medicine*, the implementation of a simple 19-item check-lists resulted in fewer complications and a 40 % drop in death rates at eight medical centers worldwide [16].

Public Versus Private Transparency

These days, the public expects quality transparency; payers are demanding it and everyone from private industries to news organizations are clamoring to set up systems to provide it. If the healthcare industry does not lead this new era, a potentially less competent third party will.

The question is not what information will be made public, but who will control that information. It is therefore important to understand the distinction—and distinct uses—of public versus private transparency.

Public physician performance transparency gives patients aggregated data that empowers them to make informed choices about their providers. Private transparency digs much deeper, giving providers the technical, granular details that can help them to evolve and improve their own performance.

Public transparency is happening all around us, from word-of-mouth recommendations by friends to online reviews to news stories about physician performance in mainstream media. Unfortunately, much of this public transparency is inaccurate, incomplete, and misleading.

In 2015 for instance, investigative journalism site ProPublica published the "Surgeon Scorecard," which used Medicare data to calculate "Adjusted Complication Rates" for surgeons performing eight in-hospital surgical procedures. These included unblinded, surgeon-level performance [17].

The scorecard found complication rates varied wildly among different providers, a finding that would give any patient pause.

The Rand Corporation ran a critique of the public transparency report, calling into question the journalists' methodology and the report's validity. In particular, the Rand Corporation highlighted the journalists' failure to properly adjust for patient risk factors and variations in hospitals' resources [18].

While many physicians and medical experts applauded ProPublica's efforts to provide patients with a physician quality transparency tool, several were quite critical of the site's methodology, including Dr. Peter Pronovost, senior vice president for patient safety and quality and director of the Armstrong Institute for Patient Safety and Quality at Johns Hopkins Medicine, who noted:

> The ProPublica measure is not valid. Though the methodology does account for some of the potential biases that might unjustly influence findings, it fails to account for another significant bias. For the ProPublica method to be a valid measure of surgical quality, all patients facing a potential readmission should have the same probability of being readmitted. Only then could readmission rates serve as a surrogate for complication rates and thus surgeon quality [19].

The journalism site retorted that its scorecard "intentionally focused on simpler elective procedures with very low complication rates and patients that were generally healthy" [20]. But clearly the questions raised underscore that there is sometimes a fine line between data that are useful to consumers and helpful to physicians and data that are harmful and irresponsible.

"A valid performance report can drive quality improvement and usefully inform patients' choices of providers. However, performance reports with poor validity and reliability are potentially damaging to all involved," the Rand Corporation wrote [18].

For public data to be truly useful, it must be comprehensive and industry-vetted. That is vetted, not censored. Collaborating with stakeholders ensures a more robust methodology that accurately reflects the reality of healthcare today.

Only slightly less controversial is private transparency. Also known as "performance feedback reports," health plans and medical groups use performance transparency internally to improve quality of care.

While little research has been done on the effectiveness of private transparency, the work that has been done has found that confidential reporting enables clinicians to assess their performance relative to peers, benchmarks, and evidence-based practice guidelines. The goal is to motivate providers to improve their performance relative to their own past efforts and to their peers—thus elevating the standard of care for all [21].

In order to be most effective, private reports should also provide doctors with access to improvement tools and resources, according to the Agency for Healthcare Research and Quality, which has studied private transparency [22].

Both public transparency and private transparency have the potential to guide innovation and improve the entire healthcare industry by revealing healthcare's needless errors, costs, and deaths. With the health system ailing, it is important to remember the old adage: Sunlight is the best disinfectant. With finely calibrated algorithms, data scientists are working to create public and private transparency tools that will result in a safer, better healthcare system.

How Performance Transparency Improves Quality of Care

U.S. healthcare spending is out of control. In 2010 healthcare spending represented 17.7 % of GDP, compared to the OECD average of 9.5 % [23, 24]. Medical costs are a significant driver of personal bankruptcies [25].

Yet, according to a 2015 Yale University study [26], the United States is not getting what it pays for in terms of healthcare quality. In a study of 19 developed nations, the United States has the highest rate of deaths from conditions that could have been prevented or treated. U.S. patients receive only about half of the care recommended for their condition, and nearly 30 % of the care delivered each year is for services that may not improve their health. The Yale study notes:

> Despite significant consequences of uninformed consumption of healthcare, evidence suggests that healthcare consumers do not spend much time determining the price and the quality of their healthcare options. But for the most part it is not because they do not want to—it is because they cannot [26].
>   In a Kaiser Family Foundation phone survey of 1517 respondents, 64 % stated that it is difficult to find information comparing the cost of different treatments and procedures offered by different doctors and hospitals [27].

Researchers argue (quite effectively) that by shedding light on what it is, exactly, that consumers are paying for, treatments will become more relevant, effective and affordable [28].

In particular, study after study has shown that quality transparency motivates health providers to change their internal policies, while enabling consumers to make informed decisions about which providers to select. And quality transparency can also have a positive effect on a health system's bottom line; hospitals that go up in their ranking by the U.S. News and World Report see an increase in non-emergency patient volume and revenue—thanks to the perception that those are "quality" institutions [29–31].

As it has in industries as varied as automotive and food manufacturing, performance transparency in healthcare elevates the entire system—lowering costs, improving quality, and creating the kind of healthy "competition" between doctors that drives innovation and excellence.

Where healthcare can improve:

- An estimated 440,000 a year die from preventable errors made during hospital stays, including treatments that should have been given but were not [32].
- As many as 11,000 deaths could have been prevented between 2010 and 2012 if patients who went to the lowest-volume hospitals had gone to the highest-volume instead [33].
- Wound infection is the leading cause of hospital readmission, affecting about 167,000 patients a year [34].

These are simple examples of areas where performance transparency can help to make quality metrics visible to consumers, help to create competition between physicians to provide better care, and help to improve overall quality.

That competition will benefit patients by matching them to the providers who are most appropriate for them. Using experience as the foundation for quality, data scientists are working to create physician performance quality scores that weigh number of cases performed, as well as the variety and severity of those cases, to offer recommendations to meet particular patients' needs.

As it is now, patients generally do not know what they are "buying" when they walk into a doctor's office or a hospital. Unless a knee replacement patient drills doctors about their experience, he would not know if they have performed 1000 knee replacements or five.

Physician performance transparency empowers patients to choose providers who are best suited to their needs, have the most experience with a particular procedure and are most likely to lead to a positive outcome and lower medical costs.

What Does It Take to Make Physician Performance Transparency a Reality?

We have now seen that physician performance transparency is a key factor in lowering the cost and increasing the quality of healthcare in the United States. But making such transparency a reality will take a confluence of great forces—patients, policy-makers, and economic models all dedicated to driving progress forward.

Consumer Demand

Patients are often puzzled by healthcare. Open enrollment periods in particular are marked by confusion and misinformation. Patients are asked to choose primary care physicians without being given enough information to make a decision that "fits" them and their families. Overwhelmed by options and underwhelmed by meaningful information, patients often base their choices on little more than a surname and a photograph.

If consumers are given access to user-friendly, factual methods for choosing quality providers, they will take advantage of them. Research out of Yale found that when information is presented in a clear, concise format, a preponderance of patients make the high-quality healthcare choice [26]. Unfortunately, that is not currently how information is presented—if it is presented at all.

Here hospitals and health systems have an opportunity to do more than list their awards on their websites. They can drill deep and offer patients the real information they want to know: Which orthopedic surgeon should I go to for my hip replacement? Which one of your neurosurgeons has the most expertise with pituitary tumors? Presented clearly and concisely, healthcare information can help consumers make better choices.

The information that is available is often not useful enough to help consumers make informed decisions. In 2015, the Kaiser Family Foundation found that 31 % of consumers report seeing information comparing doctors, hospital, and health insurance plans in the past 12 months, but only 1 in 5 recall seeing any information that offers comparisons based on quality [35].

Consumer advocacy groups and consumer-industry coalitions are agitating for exactly this level of granular data, including the Clear Choices Campaign, a consumer-industry group that includes AARP, several health insurance providers, the National Council for Behavioral Health, and others.

According to the Clear Choices Campaign: "More and better healthcare choices mean nothing if consumers don't have the tools to make informed decisions" [36].

Government Support

In 2006, President Bush signed an Executive Order to increase the transparency of the healthcare system in the United States [27]. The Executive Order directed federal agencies that administered or sponsored federal health insurance programs to increase transparency in both pricing and quality, encourage adoption of health information technology standards, and provide options that promote quality and efficiency in healthcare. A press release announcing the order explained:

> To spend their healthcare dollars wisely, Americans need to know their options in advance, know the quality of doctors and hospitals in their area, and know what procedures will cost. When Americans buy new cars, they have access to consumer research on safety, reliability, price, and performance—and they should be able to expect the same when they purchase healthcare [27].

In the intervening years, progress in physician performance transparency has been halting and inconsistent. Patients still do not have the same access to safety information for their doctors that they do for their new cars.

Government support is helping to move transparency in the right direction. Healthcare.gov and state-based health insurance exchange websites are beefing up the amount and type of information they provide consumers. And the CMS Physician Compare site now lists physician performance data for those physicians who elected to provide it.

But these are baby-steps. While the CMS reported that it had paid more than $380 million in incentive payments through its physician-quality reporting system and electronic-prescribing programs, more than 400,000 providers shrugged off the extra money—and some even accepted penalties, figuring incentives were not worth the trouble of participating [27]. As of the end of 2015, only 6 in 10 providers participated in the program [38]. Clearly much more needs to be done to incentivize and require performance transparency.

Business Models

The economics of quality care is clear. Health systems benefit from lower readmission rates, fewer ancillary procedures, and a decrease in the severity of cases as patients receive better, more appropriate preventative care.

As provider organizations begin to offer risk-based services, such as health plans, bundled payments, and ACOs, the goals between the patient, provider, and payer are becoming more aligned. This will cause quality to go up and costs to go down—but only in a world of physician performance transparency.

Physician leaders recognize that in order to make smarter business decisions, they need better information about the quality of their peers. According to a survey of providers by the American Association for Physician Leadership and the Navigant Center for Healthcare Research and Policy Analysis, 78 % of physicians described knowledge in evaluating risks associated with acquisitions or new businesses as "important or very important" [39]. In order to evaluate risks, they need data.

Finding high-quality, low-risk providers will be as important to a system's financial health as it is to the health of the patients in its care. Precise algorithms that gauge patient–doctor interactions, expertise, and other elements vital to positive healthcare outcomes, will help health systems align with "good" doctors who offer "good" care.

Conclusion

We have seen countless times in medicine that the right tools can lead to seemingly miraculous changes. Laparoscopic technology led to minimally invasive heart surgery. Our understanding of genomics is resulting in targeted cancer therapies. Just as these advances transform the capabilities of medicine, so, too, can the healthcare industry use scientifically derived advances to transform healthcare delivery.

Instead of laparoscopes or genome mapping, of course, the tool that will lead this transformation is information.

By throwing back the curtain on quality measures, big data is poised to elevate the delivery of healthcare in this nation. To effectively improve healthcare delivery, the industry needs to shift toward safer, evidenced-based, quality care. Healthcare needs to become more efficient, with fewer readmissions and unnecessary procedures. And care should be patient-centered, with well-informed consumers empowered to take a leading role in the direction of their own care.

All of that is possible, but only with proper information.

That is what makes physician performance transparency so exciting. The entire healthcare industry stands to benefit from more and more useful information about physician performance and quality. Physicians will use performance information to improve their own practices. Health systems can turn quantifiable data into actionable information that will allow them to make smarter business decisions and gain a competitive advantage.

And, of course, patients will be able to use an improved system of physician performance transparency to find the most appropriate providers for them. This will result in better outcomes and more satisfied patients.

Performance is defined as the execution of a plan. The plan for all of us—health providers, health systems, and patients alike—is to transform healthcare for the better. The key to that transformation is transparency.

References

1. Goodrich K. CMS quality measure development plan supporting the transition to the merit-based incentive payment system (MIPS) and alternative payment models (APMs) [Internet]. 2015. Available at https://blog.cms.gov/2016/05/02/cms-finalizes-its-quality-measure-development-plan/.
2. Center for Healthcare Transparency Innovation Pilot White Paper: increasing transparency on the relative cost and quality of healthcare. Portland, Maine; 2015.
3. http://www.healthcare-informatics.com/news-item/report-projects-105-million-will-be-covered-acos-2020?page=10&utm_source=feedburner&utm_medium=feed&utm_campaign=Feed%3A%20healthcare-informatics%20(Healthcare%20Informatics).
4. American Hospital Association, McManis Consulting. From volume to value: the transition to Accountable Care Organizations. White Paper; April 2011.
5. Michtalik H. Use of provider-level dashboards and pay-for-performance in venous thrombo-embolism prophylaxis. J Hosp Med. 2015;10(3):172–8.
6. http://www.ncbi.nlm.nih.gov/pubmed/21471478.
7. https://downloads.cms.gov/cmsgov/archived-downloads/SMDL/downloads/SMD073108.pdf.
8. Mehtsun WT, Ibrahim AM, Diener-West M, Pronovost PJ, Makary MA. Surgical never events in the United States. Surgery. 2013;153:465–72.
9. http://www.healthcostinstitute.org/files/2014%20HCCUR%2010.29.15.pdf.
10. www.hospitalsafetyscore.org/newsroom/display/hospitalerrors-thirdleading-causeofdeathinus-improvementstooslow.
11. http://www.ahrq.gov/professionals/quality-patient-safety/pfp/interimhacrate2014.html.
12. http://www.nationalacademies.org/hmd/Global/News%20Announcements/Crossing-the-Quality-Chasm-The-IOM-Health-Care-Quality-Initiative.aspx.
13. Porter ME. What is value in health care? N Engl J Med. 2010;363:2477–81.
14. http://www.ama-assn.org/sub/advocacy-update/2015-12-17.html.
15. Montemurro F, Mittica G, Cagnazzo C, Longo V, Berchialla P, Solinas G, et al. Self-evaluation of adjuvant chemotherapy-related adverse effects by patients with breast cancer. JAMA Oncol. 2016;2(4):445–52.
16. http://www.ajmc.com/conferences/aha2015/ticagrelor-results-suggest-patients-decide-whats-a-serious-event.
17. Haynes AB, Weiser TG, Berry W, et al. A surgical safety checklist to reduce morbidity and mortality in a global population. N Engl J Med. 2009;360:491–9.
18. https://projects.propublica.org/surgeons/.
19. http://www.rand.org/pubs/perspectives/PE170.html.
20. https://www.propublica.org/article/surgeon-level-risk-quotes.
21. https://www.propublica.org/article/our-rebuttal-to-rands-critique-of-surgeon-scorecard.
22. Kiefe C, Allison JJ, Williams OD, Person SD, Weaver MT, Weissman NW. Improving quality improvement using achievable benchmarks for physician feedback: a randomized controlled trial. JAMA. 2001;285(22):2871–9.
23. http://www.ahrq.gov/professionals/clinicians-providers/resources/privfeedbackgdrpt/privfeedbackgdrptex1-2.html.
24. http://data.worldbank.org/indicator/SH.XPD.TOTL.ZS/.
25. Centers for Medicare and Medicaid Services, Office of the Actuary, "National Health Expenditures Web Tables". Available at http://www.cms.hhs.gov/NationalHealthExpendData/downloads/tables.pdf. Accessed 3 Feb 2010.
26. http://www.pnhp.org/new_bankruptcy_study/Bankruptcy-2009.pdf.
27. Russell A. Moving the needle: how transparency could lower costs and improve quality in the United States. Harvey M. Appelbaum'59 Award 2015; paper 7. http//elischolar.library.yale.edu/appelbaum_award/7.
28. http://kff.org/health-reform/poll-finding/2008-update-on-consumers-views-of-patient-2/.

29. Marshall MN. The public release of performance data: what do we expect to gain? A review of the evidence. JAMA. 2000;283(14):1866–74.
30. Wu KH. Evaluation of the effectiveness of peer pressure to change disposition decisions and patient throughput by emergency physician. Am J Emerg Med. 2013;31(3):535–9.
31. AARP. Public comment on the release of physician data. Available at https://www.cms.gov/research-statistics-data-and-systems/statistics-trends-and-reports/medicare-provider-charge-data/downloads/publiccomments.pdf.
32. Pope D. Reacting to rakings: evidence from "America's Best Hospitals". J Health Eco. 2009. Available at http://faculty.chicagobooth.edu/devin.pope/research/pdf/website_hospitals.pdf.
33. http://www.bmj.com/content/353/bmj.i2139.
34. http://www.nejm.org/doi/full/10.1056/NEJMsa0903048.
35. http://media.jamanetwork.com/news-item/hospital-readmissions-after-surgery-associated-mostly-with-complications-related-to-surgical-procedure/.
36. http://kff.org/health-costs/poll-finding/kaiser-health-tracking-poll-april-2015/.
37. http://www.clearchoicescampaign.org/.
38. http://www.modernhealthcare.com/article/20150424/NEWS/150429944.
39. https://www.cms.gov/Medicare/Quality-Initiatives-Patient-Assessment-Instruments/PQRS/AnalysisAndPayment.html.

Chapter 4
Assuring Appropriate Care

Charles E. Coffey Jr. and Teryl K. Nuckols

Introduction

To improve healthcare delivery, one must first know what care should and should not be delivered to a specific patient, for a given set of conditions, at a specific time, and in a specific setting or location. That is, healthcare providers, leaders, and change agents must be comfortable with defining appropriate care, and then designing systems to both ensure patients receive appropriate care and to prevent the delivery of inappropriate care.

Unexplained Variation in Clinical Practice

In 2014, the United States spent $3.0 trillion, or 17.5 %, of its gross domestic product on healthcare costs [1]. Despite the huge amount of money spent on healthcare, the US rates poorly in many health outcomes, including life expectancy and prevalence of chronic diseases [2]. Looking more closely at healthcare spending and related outcomes, researchers have identified large variations in healthcare spending by region of the country with little to no variation in the

C.E. Coffey Jr., M.D., M.S., F.H.M., F.A.C.P. (✉)
Los Angeles County + University of Southern California Medical Center,
2051 Marengo Street, C2K100, Los Angeles, CA 90033, USA
e-mail: CCoffeyJr@DHS.LACounty.gov

T.K. Nuckols
Department of Medicine, Cedars Sinai Medical Center,
8700 Beverly Blvd; Becker Building, Suite 100, Los Angeles, CA 90048, USA

© Springer International Publishing Switzerland 2017   41
H.C. Sax (ed.), *Measurement and Analysis in Transforming Healthcare Delivery*, DOI 10.1007/978-3-319-46222-6_4

outcomes of care [3] or satisfaction with care [4]. The variations in care delivery are widespread across settings and clinical conditions, and impact both medical and surgical-based specialties. Even the lay press has picked up on the widespread variation in care delivery and associated variation in care delivery cost. For example, The New Yorker published a pair of articles describing the discrepancies in cost and outcomes in two cities in Texas, McAllen and El Paso, by renowned surgeon and author, Atul Gawande [5, 6]. With the growing body of medical and lay literature demonstrating that variation in healthcare delivery results in variation in healthcare cost, healthcare leaders and policy makers alike recognize that, if the US is going to bend the cost curve of healthcare, it must eliminate unwarranted variation in clinical practice.

While some care delivery varies in cost, other care delivery varies by the overuse or underuse of care. For example, McGlynn and colleagues found that U.S. adults received only 50–60 % of recommended care regardless of whether the care type was preventative care, acute care, or care of chronic conditions [7]. In that study, underuse of care was detected among 46.3 % of patients (meaning they were not offered highly beneficial care), while overuse was found among 11.3 % (meaning they received potentially harmful care). In addition, Lawson and colleagues observed both overuse and underuse of surgical care across 16 of the most commonly performed surgical procedures [8].

Health systems and payers are seeking to rein in costs by reducing the unexplained variation in care delivery, and to improve quality of care by addressing underuse and overuse. The development and application of criteria to determine appropriate care is one key tool payers and health systems are using to accomplish the goal of reducing unwarranted variation in care delivery and cost. Developing appropriateness criteria forces providers, payers, and health systems to agree to what type of care is and is not warranted in a clinical scenario and/or clinical setting. Given the growing importance of appropriateness criteria by payers and health systems, it is critical that physicians understand how to define appropriateness, how appropriateness criteria are developed, and most importantly, how to use appropriateness criteria to improve care delivery.

The Various Conceptualizations of Appropriateness

In their seminal work, Brook, Chasin, and colleagues defined appropriate care as care delivered to the patient where the benefits of the care (test, procedure, medication, etc.) exceed the risks involved in receiving that care, irrespective of cost [9]. Conversely, care is considered inappropriate when the risks to the patient exceed the potential benefits [9]. Although this definition is simple, the various stakeholders in the healthcare system—clinicians, patients, payers, and health systems—have different perspectives on how to define appropriateness. This section will discuss the various definitions of appropriateness for each stakeholder.

The Physician

Many physicians are likely to think of appropriate care as care that improves clinical outcomes. When conceptualizing the care that would be appropriate for an individual patient, physicians are able to draw on a combination of published evidence as well as knowledge gained from years of clinical practice [10]. How physicians think of appropriateness, however, may have shifted in recent years. Physicians may be increasingly considering additional factors, including patient preference, patient satisfaction, and perhaps also cost to the patient and health system. Groups like the Institute of Medicine are placing greater emphasis on delivering care that is patient-centered, meaning care that takes into account the patients "preferences, needs, and values and ensuring that patient values guide all clinical decisions" [11]. Furthermore, shifts away from fee-for-service reimbursement models and toward value-based reimbursement models often involve holding physicians accountable for patient satisfaction and the cost of care. Reconciling these disparate issues in day-to-day practice poses challenges for physicians because what may make a patient happy may not yield the best clinical outcome or may come at a higher cost. Indeed, a 2012 study found that higher patient satisfaction was associated with increased mortality as well as higher overall healthcare expenditures [12]. Physicians face "catch 22" scenarios regularly, such as responding to patient requests for early imaging of low back pain, when such imaging leads to more surgery and illness "labeling" without offering health benefits [13].

The Healthcare Payer

Payers have a practical need to define appropriate care because they must make determinations about which clinical services to reimburse for which patients. Often, payers establish medical necessity standards, and define care as appropriate when it meets those standards. For example, in on-line materials, Cigna has defined care as medically necessary if the "healthcare services that a [p]hysician, exercising prudent clinical judgment, would provide to a patient for the purpose of evaluating, diagnosing or treating an illness, injury, disease or its symptoms, and that are:

- In accordance with the generally accepted standards of medical practice;
- Clinically appropriate, in terms of type, frequency, extent, site and duration, and considered effective for the patient's illness, injury or disease; and
- Not primarily for the convenience of the patient or [p]hysician, or other [p]hysician, and not more costly than an alternative service or sequence of services at least as likely to produce equivalent therapeutic or diagnostic results as to the diagnosis or treatment of that patient's illness, injury or disease" [14].

Payers also consider the setting of care delivery when determining if care is appropriate, because, as Lavis and Anderson argue, care should be delivered in the most cost-effective setting while still being effective and safe [15]. Criteria for assessing the appropriateness of the care delivery setting are typically independent of the diagnosis, and are applicable to most categories of patients. For example, a screening colonoscopy is most cost-effective if done in an outpatient setting like an outpatient procedure center or endoscopy suite. From the payer's perspective, aligning appropriate care with the appropriate care delivery setting is fundamental to ensuring that care is delivered in an efficient and cost-effective manner.

The Patient

When conceptualizing appropriate care, patients are likely to weigh perceived benefits and risks, financial obligations determined by their health insurance coverage and benefits, convenience, and personal beliefs and preferences. Patients have varying degrees of medical knowledge and health literacy that may influence their understanding of potential benefits and risks. The Internet gives patients easy access to medical information of variable quality as well as the opinions of other patients. Direct-to-consumer marketing makes patients more aware of expensive new medications, tests, and treatment options. Individuals may also perceive the potential risks and benefits of care differently due to historical and cultural factors as well as religious affiliations. Increasingly, patients are faced with higher insurance premiums, deductibles, and other forms of cost sharing. Consequently, financial obligations may be more burdensome for some patients today than it was in the past.

The Researcher

Although initially developed for research purposes, the definition of appropriateness set forth by Brook and his colleagues in the RAND/UCLA Appropriateness Method is generally well aligned with the physician, payer, and patient perspectives, although there are areas of potential disagreement [9]. Based on clinical risks and benefits, irrespective of cost, Brook et al. places care into four categories: necessary care (benefits greatly exceed risks such that it must be offered), appropriate care (benefits greatly exceed risks), care of uncertain appropriateness, and inappropriate care (risks exceed benefits to such a degree that it should not be provided) [9]. Ensuring patients receive care that provides benefit while minimizing or avoiding harm aligns with the payers' objective of ensuring medical necessity and the physician and patients' desires for the best possible clinical outcome [9].

Payers are likely to support defining potentially harmful care as inappropriate care, but may have a different perception of care that Brook et al. would classify as of uncertain appropriateness. The RAND/UCLA Appropriateness Method makes no statements about whether or not care of uncertain appropriateness should be provided. Yet much of the healthcare provided to patients today is likely to be classified as of uncertain appropriateness due to limitations to clinical evidence and variations in patients' clinical circumstances. Payers are generally more willing to cover care for which appropriateness is well established than care of uncertain appropriateness. However, they still need to make coverage determinations in such situations—determinations that require subjective and potentially challenging judgments that can lead to disputes with physicians and patients. By requiring consideration of less costly alternatives or lower cost settings, payers can reduce costs without issuing a denial of coverage.

Regarding care of uncertain appropriateness, patients' views may sometimes conflict with those of payers. Whereas payers would prefer to cover care for which clinical benefits are well established, some patients may expect coverage for any care that they personally believe to offer some possibility of benefit. Some patients may be disappointed that healthcare payers choose not to cover unproven herbal remedies, for example.

Developing and Applying Appropriateness Criteria

As discussed above, key healthcare stakeholders can have different definitions of appropriateness. These stakeholders also have different ways of applying the appropriateness criteria to influence care delivery. This section discusses how physicians, payers, health systems, and healthcare researchers develop and apply appropriateness criteria to care delivery.

Developing and Applying Appropriateness Criteria: An Overview

There are three key elements to developing and applying appropriateness criteria: a literature review, evaluation of the criteria by clinical experts, and implementation. The literature review serves as the foundation for clinical reasoning. The quality of the literature review methods used to develop appropriateness criteria and the extent of the evidence base can vary, potentially affecting credibility to physicians. Having subject matter experts in the relevant clinical fields review, modify, and vote on the criteria can help to fill gaps in the evidence base, assess feasibility and applicability of the appropriateness criteria to specific clinical settings, and determine whether the criteria are aligned with current standards of practice. Once appropriateness criteria are developed, the next step is implementation. Criteria can be adopted nationally, such as by major healthcare payers, or adopted by local communities of physicians and healthcare delivery settings. During the process of implementation, adjustment, revision, and adaptation can help to ensure that local stakeholders view the criteria as credible and that the criteria are aligned with local care delivery patterns. Thus, the adoption and concurrent adaptation process may modify the criteria, but ultimately, this allows for better implementation and, hopefully, adherence.

Developing and Applying Appropriateness Criteria: The Physician

Physicians and physician groups participate in developing appropriateness criteria for two main reasons: (1) To ensure the criteria are consistent with physicians' style of practice when linking care, quality, and value, and (2) To develop practice guidelines to assist physicians at the point of care when caring for patients.

As payers, including the Centers for Medicare and Medicaid (CMS), use appropriateness criteria to rein in costs and standardize care, they are becoming more prescriptive in defining appropriateness criteria. For example, with the passage of the Medicare Access and CHIP Reauthorization Act of 2015, the U.S. Congress created a new framework for CMS to reward physicians for quality of care [16]. The framework for defining high value care that CMS will reimburse has yet to be defined. Consequently, physicians and physician groups see an opportunity to create appropriateness of care standards that more closely match existing practice patterns rather than being forced to adopt a different, and possibly stricter, set of criteria developed and adopted by CMS and other payers.

The second reason physicians and physician groups develop appropriateness criteria is to assist physicians in caring for patients. For clinicians, developing appropriateness criteria starts with a thorough understanding of the medical literature. Indeed, the complex task of determining appropriate care for the patient is simplified if there are concrete, well-defined, and actionable criteria for specific patients and/or choices for testing and treatment defined in the medical literature [15]. Randomized control trials, however, are often limited in their generalizability, and due to the cost and time it takes to conduct a randomized control trial, there simply are not enough trials completed to develop appropriateness criteria for every possible clinical scenario. To guide decision-making in scenarios where research is limited, physicians rely on other forms of knowledge, including expert consensus opinion statements and clinical practice guidelines. Indeed, many prominent physician groups develop and promote appropriateness criteria and related clinical practice guidelines for their specialty.

Physicians use two mechanisms to adopt and adapt of these criteria to their local practice environment. The first mechanism of adoption and adaptation is the use of these standards in creating and/or revising care delivery pathways at the local institution. For example, a physician may use the newest version of the American College of Chest Physician's peri-operative anticoagulation practice guidelines to update workflows and order sets at the local hospital. The second mechanism of adoption and adaptation is the participation in Utilization Management (UM) structures at the local institution. As part of a joint effort between the payer, the physicians, and the local healthcare system, the UM process allows physicians to participate in the application of appropriateness standards to clinical case reviews. Through participation with UM, physicians can use their clinical knowledge and expertise in case reviews while also promoting adherence to appropriateness standards.

Developing and Applying Appropriateness Criteria: The Payer and the Health System

Payers, hospitals, and health systems use third-party appropriateness criteria developed from the same three-step process used by physicians. These companies include groups like the Professional Standards Review Organization and their Appropriateness Evaluation Protocol (AEP), InterQual and the Intensity-Severity-Discharge Appropriateness (ISD-A), and Milliman and the Milliman Care Guidelines (MCG). Each set of guidelines are developed by a process of literature review and consensus building by using physicians and nurses retrospectively reviewing clinical cases, and both the AEP and ISD-A have been validated by comparing these criteria with assessments of appropriateness of setting done by panels of physicians [15, 17, 18]. All the guidelines describe appropriateness of care criteria for outpatient and hospital-based care, and all the guidelines are kept up to date routinely through annual literature reviews.

The appropriateness criteria can be applied in both a prospective and retrospective manner. Payers, hospitals, and health systems apply these criteria prospectively through the prior authorization process. This process allows the insurer to review a proposed test or treatment for a patient and the given clinical context, and prior to the patient undergoing the test or treatment, offer a judgment of appropriate use. If the test or treatment is appropriate given the clinical context, the payer will agree to pay the hospital or health system for the service rendered; if judged as inappropriate, the payer will not pay for the service.

There is a two-phase retrospective application of appropriateness guidelines by the payer and the hospital or health system to determine if care delivered is appropriate. First, the hospital or health system applies the guidelines by comparing the models' criteria to the patient's current severity of illness and intensity of service needs for that day as determined by chart review [15]. This review is often done by a UM nurse or physician advisor, and based on this review, the hospital or health system can request reimbursement for services rendered by submitting a bill to the payer. If the reviewer identifies a part of the patient's care that may not meet the appropriateness standards, the reviewer will work with the responsible physician to understand the case further and justify the resource utilization. Second, the payer applies the same criteria to the chart for their own appropriateness assessment. Should the payer find the care appropriate, it will pay the hospital or health system for the service rendered. Should the payer find there was inappropriate use of resources upon retrospective review of patient charts, the payer can deny reimbursement to the hospital or health system for that service rendered.

Although these models are effective for determining appropriateness of inpatient services, they have three major limitations. First, some of the models cannot determine appropriateness of care delivered after the patient leaves the hospital [15]. For example, neither the AEP or ISD-A models extend to care delivered in long-term care facilities or at home with home health services; the MCG model does include criteria for home care and recovery facilities [19]. Second, the models assume that the level and mix of healthcare providers are constant, and so fail to determine appropriateness of resources used during the day of hospitalization [15]. That is, while the models may deem a hospital day appropriate, there may be a multitude of unnecessary services rendered to the patient during that appropriate hospital day, independent of the actual service need that determined the patient was appropriate for hospitalization. Lastly, the models are used most often in a retrospective manner after the care has been delivered. Hospital UM departments, though, are moving toward a real-time review process so as to prevent inappropriate or unnecessary services from being delivered in the first place, or even identify patients who may need a given service while hospitalized, thus preventing both overuse and underuse of resources [15].

Developing and Applying Appropriateness Criteria: The Researcher

To produce effective and useful clinical research on appropriateness of care, researchers need clear and precise definitions of appropriateness. As such, the best appropriateness criteria for research are comprehensive, developed by a multi-disciplinary group, and applicable to most clinical situations [10]. The most well-known method for developing appropriateness criteria for research is the RAND/UCLA appropriateness method (RAM). The RAND Corporation is a public policy think tank and research institute that developed a methodology to define appropriateness criteria using a combination of evidence from the medical literature and expert consensus opinion for treatment of seven specific medical and surgical services, including coronary artery bypass graft (CABG), coronary angiography, percutaneous transluminal coronary angioplasty, carotid endarterectomy, hysterectomy, and placement of tympanostomy tubes [9].

The RAND/UCLA method of defining appropriateness starts with conducting an extensive synthesis of the medical literature for the best evidence for and against treatment of a given condition. Next, the researchers select a panel of nine physicians, representing different clinical specialties (e.g., Cardiology, Internal Medicine, Surgery) and the various regions of the country. Using the literature review as shared foundation of medical knowledge, the individual panel members rank independently the appropriateness of the treatment for a patient given specific clinical conditions proposed by the researchers. The panel then meets, discusses all the relevant medical literature, and reviews the blinded ratings of all panelists for each of the clinical scenarios. After this review and discussion process, the panelists rate the indications a second time, and finalize the set of appropriateness criteria for a specific service (e.g., CABG) given various clinical scenarios [9]. These criteria can then be applied in research studies to assess if care is or is not appropriate.

The RAND Corporation first published their method for developing appropriateness criteria in 1991. Since then, researchers have studied its methodology extensively. Shekelle summarized a review of this research on RAM and found that the RAM has an estimated sensitivity between 68 and 99 % and an estimated specificity between 94 and 97 % [10]. In addition, Shekelle notes that studies have shown that the RAM criteria are very sensitive to the makeup of the panel and the influence of the moderator, but the RAM criteria are reproducible if the clinical disciplines of panel composition is held constant [10]. Although appropriateness criteria developed using the RAM method are reproducible, sensitive and specific, it is a costly and time-consuming process, and the criteria must be updated on a frequent and regular basis as new literature is published. Shekelle argues, though, that researchers and clinicians can overcome the time and cost barriers by leveraging technology [10]. For example, compiling, synthesizing, and sharing the literature can be done via e-mail; subject matter expert panel meetings can be held virtually; voting on the criteria can be done using new programs or applications for the computer, tablet, or smartphone. Despite the advantages of RAM, and the advances in technology since it was first published back in 1991, the health systems and payer organizations have been slow to use RAM to develop and implement appropriateness criteria.

The History of Appropriateness Criteria

Physicians have long considered appropriateness of care when practicing medicine. Indeed, the concept of appropriateness is central to the practice of evidence-based medicine. Yet prior to the birth of Medicare and Medicaid, there was wide practice variation between physicians caring for similar types of patients. In the 1950s and early 1960s, there were few practice guidelines and little focus on utilization management. Consequently, physicians relied on best common practices and their own clinical judgment to ensure patients received the best clinical care [20]. Through the Social Security Act of 1965, the United States Congress created Medicare and Medicaid, and in doing so, made the United States Federal government a major payer of healthcare services. Along with the implementation of Medicare and Medicaid, the government also instituted various controls on healthcare spending and resource utilization. As a consequence, health systems had to review how they cared for patients, including hospitals, which were now required to review each patient admission for medical necessity, hospital length of stay, and resource utilization during the hospitalization [20]. Furthermore, Medicare and Medicaid started issuing retrospective payment denials for inappropriate services rendered. The combination of requirement for utilization review and retrospective payment denials made appropriateness assessments and utilization management critical to the financial success of healthcare organizations.

To help healthcare organizations conduct utilization reviews, and to avoid payment denials, organizations like the Commission on Hospital and Professional Activities (CHPA) developed utilization guidelines and case mix index norms by analyzing historical patient data. One of the first such set of guidelines was the Professional Activity Study (PAS) from the CHPA. The PAS guidelines outlined case mix index, the process of treatment, and certain clinical outcomes for most regions of the country [21, 22]. The PAS guidelines, however, were insufficient because they were built on a limited sample of patient cases from regional hospitals, lacked specificity, and were difficult to apply to the care of the patient [20, 22]. Consequently, new companies like InterQual developed more clinically relevant utilization guidelines based on severity of illness and resource utilization. These guidelines further aligned appropriate care with appropriate resource utilization. By the early 1980s, InterQual became the preferred source of appropriateness guidelines for intensity of service based on severity of illness.

Appropriateness of service became even more important to the financial health of hospitals with the introduction of the Inpatient Prospective Payment System (IPSS) in 1983. With the IPSS, Medicare used Diagnosis-Related Groups (DRG) to establish expected intensity of service and related hospital reimbursement rates for a given patient. Under the DRG reimbursement system Medicare pays hospitals a flat fee for the care of a patient with a given DRG [23]. Consequently, to maximize their profit on providing care for Medicare patients for a flat reimbursement fee, hospitals must ensure appropriate resource use.

Despite the use of appropriateness criteria in Medicaid and Medicare reimbursement, healthcare spending in the United States grew exponentially over the 1990s and 2000s. By 2005, the United States spent greater than 15 % of its gross domestic product on healthcare [24]. Healthcare leaders from the private and government sectors recognized that this level of resource consumption was unsustainable, and that change was needed. In 2010, President Barack Obama signed into law the Patient Protection and Affordable Care Act, which, among other actions, ushered in a new era of payment reform for healthcare services. With the Affordable Care Act (ACA), the Federal government introduced mechanisms to change the way Medicare reimburses health systems and healthcare providers. That is, the ACA rewards coordinated, efficient and appropriate care delivery through its focus on care value rather than care volume. Specifically, the ACA allows Medicare and Medicaid to reimburse healthcare systems like Accountable Care Organizations a flat fee for care delivered for a given set of patients for a specified time frame (i.e., per member per month, or capitation). In addition, under its Hospital Acquired Complication Reduction Program, the ACA allows Medicare and Medicaid to not reimburse health systems and providers for care that occurs in response to complications of care. For example, hospitals are no longer reimbursed for care provided for a hospital-acquired complication, like *C. difficile* diarrhea. Lastly, the ACA introduces bundled payments, which allows the government to pay a set amount for a specific type of care delivered. For example, a health system and surgeon both receive a fixed rate of reimbursement for a total hip arthroplasty. This fixed reimbursement rate covers all aspects of the care for that patient's procedure, including any services rendered in the pre-operative setting, in the hospital, and after discharge. Consequently, health systems and providers are now rewarded financially to ensure that patient care is appropriate, both in terms of the actual care delivered and the setting in which that care is delivered. This collection of incentives and penalties that is aligning health systems and healthcare providers around the concept of appropriateness is neatly coined Value-Based Purchasing (VBP).

Although the Fee-for-Service reimbursement model still exists and is widely used, by creating new reimbursement models, the ACA realigns the financial incentives to reward healthcare delivery systems like Accountable Care Organizations (ACO) and Patient-Centered Medical Homes (PCMH) that provide efficient, appropriate care. Building on the changes implemented with the ACA, the Department of Health and Human Services (HHS) is now working to further tie physician and health system reimbursement to quality or value. Indeed, HHS projects that 90 % of all Medicare fee-for-service payments will be tied to quality or value by 2018. Furthermore, HHS anticipates that 50 % of Medicare fee-for-service payments will be tied to alternative payment models like ACOs and PCMHs by 2018 [25]. In addition, with the repeal of the Medicare Sustainable Growth Rate formula in 2015, the United States Congress has reinforced the linkage between Medicare reimbursement for physicians and their participation in alternative payment models like ACOs and PCMHs. Now, more than ever, to survive financially, providers and healthcare organizations must define and follow appropriateness criteria, both for the type of care delivered and the setting in which that care is delivered.

Using Appropriateness Criteria to Improve Healthcare: A Practical Guide

There are numerous opportunities to improve the delivery of appropriate care. For example, physicians working in the hospital setting may use the InterQual admission criteria to evaluate the appropriateness of each hospitalization. As another example, physicians may use the American College of Radiology's Appropriateness criteria to ensure patients get the best diagnostic imaging study for the clinical scenario. Physicians and health systems not using appropriateness criteria to improve the care delivery will begin feeling pressure from patients, payers, and regulators to do so soon. This section outlines a simple three-step process to help physicians and other healthcare leaders design and implement appropriateness criteria at the local level. This section also illustrates how three organizations, Cedars-Sinai Health System, InterMountain Healthcare, and the Michigan Health and Hospital Association, have used appropriateness criteria to improve care delivery at hospitals.

There are three key steps to designing and implementing care using appropriateness criteria:

1. Define appropriateness criteria for specific clinical conditions, situations, or settings of care
2. Design and implement a process (a sequence of steps or actions taken to deliver care) that ensures the delivery of appropriate care or prevent the delivery of inappropriate care
3. Design and use tools that help facilitate the care delivery process

Although there are only three steps to implementing appropriate care, the steps themselves require hard work and collaboration across many clinical disciplines. After identifying a specific opportunity to improve the appropriateness of care, the first step is to define what care is and is not appropriate. Start by searching the literature for appropriateness criteria, including both randomized control trials, meta-analyses, and guidelines and consensus statements. Table 4.1 lists several key Internet resources for you to use when starting a search for appropriateness criteria. If no clear appropriateness standards exist after the literature search, use a modified version of the RAND/UCLA Appropriateness Method to create appropriateness standards. To use the RAND/UCLA Appropriateness Method locally, start by identifying and organizing local subject matter experts (SME) and stakeholders into a panel. Next, use this panel to define the criteria for appropriate care for the specific clinical scenario needing improvement. Then have the panel review the existing care delivery processes, and associated outcomes data to determine if the care delivered at your institution is meeting the appropriateness criteria.

After defining specific appropriateness criteria, the next step is to develop and implement processes that both support the delivery of appropriate care and prevent the delivery of inappropriate care. The care delivery process is defined as a series of actions or steps taken to ensure the patient receives the intended care. Ideally, a multi-disciplinary team, including physicians, nurses, relevant staff, and patients, will either revise existing care delivery processes or develop a new process to meet the intended goal. The new process must be sure to match the right patient with the right care, and will likely leverage the electronic medical record and electronic order entry through the use of order sets, pathways, and care bundles.

Adherence to the new process is key to ensuring appropriate care is delivered. Tools like checklists, electronic reminders, and point-of-care practice alerts help ensure adherence to the new process. Measure both the rate of adherence to the process as well as the outcomes of that process, to ensure successful delivery of appropriate care. Providers, staff, and patients will want to know how the new process is working, so data transparency will be important to keep the team engaged and promote continued success. Audit and feedback of data on the performance of the process is a powerful mechanism to influence behavior and to drive change, and should be used as a tool to help communicate to others about the success of your efforts. Sharing data will also help engage others in a discussion on how to improve the new process. Adjust the process and tools accordingly to meet your goal.

Table 4.1 Internet resources for care appropriateness

Organization	Address	Description
Agency for Healthcare Research and Quality	www.AHRQ.gov	A comprehensive website for both clinicians and patients that provides evidence-based information on appropriateness of care among many other topics
American College of Radiology Appropriateness Criteria	www.acr.org/quality-safety/ appropriateness-criteria	On-line database for providers to use when determining the appropriate imaging study for a given clinical scenario
Choosing Wisely	www.ChoosingWisely.org	An initiative of the American Board of Internal Medicine Foundation, this campaign and associated website is designed to help eliminate wasteful testing, treatments and procedures
Cochrane Reviews	www.Cochrane.org	Cochrane Reviews are systematic reviews of the medical literature that focus on the accuracy of diagnostic tests along with the effects of interventions for prevention and treatment
Costs of Care	www.CostsOfCare.org	On-line resource intended to teach healthcare providers about designing and implementing high value care; it has a large focus on the cost of care
Institute for Healthcare Improvement	www.IHI.org	This website has numerous tools and tutorials around designing high value healthcare delivery processes
Lown Institute	www.LownInstitute.org	A grassroots organization seeking to improve the healthcare delivery system, with a focus on over- and underuse of testing and treatment

Case Studies

Improving the Appropriateness of Cardiac Monitoring at Cedars-Sinai Medical Center

At Cedars-Sinai Medical Center, clinicians monitor the heart rate and rhythm of majority of hospitalized patients using the cardiac monitor (CM). Providers prescribe CM for hospitalized patients often at admission, and then fail to stop CM when it no longer becomes necessary. Indeed, review of the current practice patterns revealed that majority of patients had an appropriate reason for CM upon initiation of the monitor, but once the reason for CM resolved or was treated, CM was continued without indication. Consequently, despite having 241 medical-surgical beds capable of CM, the use of CM was a bottleneck for patient flow at Cedars-Sinai, resulting in longer patient lengths of stay in the Emergency Department, intensive care units, and post-anesthesia care units. To reduce potential overuse of CM and to improve patient flow, we implemented a modified version of the 2004 American Heart Association's (AHA) appropriateness criteria for CM. After identifying the AHA CM criteria as our foundation for appropriate use of CM, we asked our local subject matter experts, including several cardiologists, to review and adapt the criteria for local use. Once the CM criteria were finalized and approved by the key medical staff and medical center governance structures, we built a process into our electronic medical record to ensure the use of these CM guidelines. Specifically, we built an order panel that required providers to indicate a clinical indication for CM for every patient. As suggested by the AHA CM guidelines, each CM criteria had an associated time limit—24-, 48-h, or until the provider discontinues the CM. We also built a supporting workflow for physicians and nursing staff to remove CM from clinically stable patients when the order expired. We used various tools, including reminders and point-of-care practice alerts, to ensure physician and nursing adherence to the new processes. To date, physicians and nurses alike have accepted evidence-based ordering and renewal cardiac monitoring, and the process has resulted in 40 % of patients experiencing time-limited cardiac monitoring [26].

Intermountain Healthcare

At InterMountain Healthcare (IMH), an integrated health system in Salt Lake City, Utah, delivering appropriate, standardized care is key to their clinical and financial success. In the mid-1980s, IMH started measuring variation in care delivered by various providers for the same clinical scenario. Through this process, the IMH leadership quickly learned that there was wide variation in care delivery for a given clinical scenario, not only between providers, but sometimes by the providers themselves. Consequently, and in order to improve the care delivered by IMH providers, the IMH leadership knew that they needed to focus on improving the care delivery processes that underlie particular treatments rather than focusing on changing provider behavior. This insight launched over 30 years' worth of work to improve the quality and value of care delivered at IMH. The first clinical scenario that IMH worked to improve was treatment of acute respiratory distress syndrome (ARDS). Alan Morris, an IMH Pulmonologist, and his team of physicians and nurses defined appropriate treatment of ARDS at IMH, and then implemented care delivery processes and tools, including care pathways and checklists, to improve the appropriateness of ARDS care at IMH. In the process, patient survival from ARDS improved from 9 to 44 % and cost of care fell by 25 % [27]. As Morris and his colleagues shared their results with their peers, IMH system leadership gleaned that this model of defining appropriate evidence-based care and designing supporting processes to ensure its delivery would be applicable to other clinical scenarios. Building off of the success from the ARDS care improvement project, IMH created an organizational structure that defined appropriate care for the 104 care processes that accounted for 95 % of IMH's care delivery, including processes for newborn deliveries, C-sections, and hip replacements. For each care process, IMH convened a group of physician and nursing SMEs to define the standard of care. In addition, these groups also developed underlying support processes to ensure all patients receive the IMH standard of care. As new literature emerged, and performance changed, these groups would reconvene and adjust the standards of care and supporting processes where necessary. IMH distributed regularly physician-level performance on adherence to this standard of care, and worked with clinicians to understand any variation that IMH observed over time. As a result of this great work, IMH has become a national leader in delivering low cost, high quality care [27].

The Michigan Health and Hospital Association Keystone ICU Project

In 2003–2004, 103 ICUs, 98 from the state of Michigan and 5 from outside of Michigan, participated in the Keystone ICU Project to reduce central line-associated blood stream infection (CLABSI) in the ICU. To create the appropriate care standards, the Keystone Project leaders bundled together 5 evidence-based interventions that had been shown to through prior research to reduce CLABSIs. The leaders then disseminated this bundle and facilitated its implementation in the ICUs. Included in the bundle were instructions to design and implement key care delivery processes, including requiring ICU teams to discuss necessity and removal of central lines on a daily basis. In addition, the bundle included key tools to facilitate adherence to the new processes, such as one checklist for daily central line care and another checklist for the development and maintenance of a central line insertion cart to ensure all supplies needed for the insertion were available. The results of the Keystone ICU project were astonishing: a significant and sustained decrease in the rates of CLABSIs for all ICUs during the study period. By defining the standards for appropriate central line care for the ICUs, and developing critical processes and tools to facilitate the delivery of the appropriate care, the Keystone ICU Project was able to improve care across 103 ICUs [28].

Chapter Summary

Appropriateness is a key concept in the evolving landscape of healthcare. With the Affordable Care Act of 2010, the United States Federal Government is aligning financial incentives and penalties to promote high-quality, appropriate care delivered efficiently and equitably. Defining appropriate care, though, can be challenging. At its core, appropriate care is care whose benefits outweigh the risks, thus making the care worth doing [10]. To help define and develop appropriateness criteria, practitioners and researchers alike can use the RAND/UCLA Appropriateness Method, or a modified version of the RAND/UCLA method, as a framework. With the shift away from fee-for-service reimbursement and toward a fee-for-value reimbursement model, one should consider the cost and setting of care in addition to clinical criteria when developing appropriateness criteria. Understanding how to define and assess appropriateness of care is important, but even more important is the effort to redesign care to improve the delivery of appropriate care and to prevent the delivery of inappropriate care. This effort must be led by physicians and nurses to be successful. We hope that following the three-step process of defining, implementing and measuring appropriateness of care delivery will help you and your team be successful in this endeavor.

References

1. National Healthcare Expenditures 2014 highlights. https://www.cms.gov/Research-Statistics-Data-and-Systems/Statistics-Trends-and-Reports/NationalHealthExpendData/Downloads/highlights.pdf. Accessed 23 April 2016.
2. Squires D, Anderson C. U.S. Health Care from a global perspective: spending, use of services, prices, and health in 13 countries. The Commonwealth Fund. 2015. Available at http://www.commonwealthfund.org/publications/issue-briefs/2015/oct/us-health-care-from-a-global-perspective. Accessed 23 April 2016.
3. Fisher ES, Wennberg DE, Stukel TA, Gottlieb MS, Lucas FL, Pinder EL. The implications of regional variations in Medicare spending part 1: the content, quality and accessibility of care. Ann Intern Med. 2003;138:273–87.
4. Fisher ES, Wennberg DE, Stukel TA, Gottlieb MS, Lucas FL, Pinder EL. The implications of regional variations in Medicare spending part 2: health outcomes and satisfaction with care. Ann Intern Med. 2003;138:288–98.
5. Gawande A. The cost conundrum. The New Yorker, 1 June 2009. Available at http://www.newyorker.com/magazine/2009/06/01/the-cost-conundrum. Accessed 19 May 2016.
6. Gawande A. Overkill. The New Yorker, 4 May 2015. Available at http://www.newyorker.com/magazine/annals-of-health-care. Accessed 19 May 2016.
7. McGlynn EA, Asch SM, Adams J, Keesey JK, Hicks J, DeCristofaro A, Kerr EA. The quality of health care delivered to adults in the United States. N Engl J Med. 2003;348:2635–45.
8. Lawson EH, Gibbons MM, Ingraham AM, Shekelle PG, Ko CY. Appropriateness criteria to assess variations in surgical procedure use in the United States. Arch Surg. 2011;146(12):1433–40.
9. Brook R, Chassin M, Fink A, Solomon D, Kosecoff J, Park R. A method for the detailed assessment of the appropriateness of medical technologies. RAND Corporation. 1991. Available at http://www.rand.org/pubs/notes/N3376.html. Accessed 19 May 2016.
10. Shekelle PG. The appropriateness method. Med Decis Making. 2004;24:228–31. doi:10.1177/0272989X04264212.
11. Institute of Medicine (U.S.). Crossing the quality chasm: a new health system for the 21st century. Washington, DC: National Academy Press; 2001.
12. Fenton JJ, Jerant AF, Bertakis KD, Franks P. The cost of satisfaction: a national study of patient satisfaction, health care utilization, expenditures, and mortality. Arch Intern Med. 2012;172(5):405–11. doi:10.1001/archinternmed.2011.1662.

13. Chou R, Qaseem A, Snow V, Casey D, Cross Jr JT, Shekelle PG, Owens DK. Diagnosis and treatment of low back pain: a joint clinical practice guideline from the American College of Physicians and the American Pain Society. Ann Intern Med. 2008;147(7):478–91.
14. Cigna. http://www.cigna.com/healthcare-professionals/resources-for-health-care-professionals/clinical-payment-and-reimbursement-policies/medical-necessity-definitions.
15. Lavis JN, Anderson GM. Appropriateness in health care delivery: definitions, measurement and policy implications. Can Med Assoc J. 1996;154(3):321–8.
16. Centers for Medicare and Medicaid Quality Payment Program. Available at https://www.cms.gov/Medicare/Quality-Initiatives-Patient-Assessment-Instruments/Value-Based-Programs/MACRA-MIPS-and-APMs/MACRA-MIPS-and-APMs.html. Accessed 19 May 2016.
17. Gertman PM, Restuccia JD. The appropriateness evaluation protocol: a technique for assessing unnecessary days of hospital care. Med Care. 1981;19:855–71.
18. McDonagh MS, Smith DH, Goddard M. Measuring appropriate use of acute beds: a systematic review of methods and results. Health Policy. 2000;53:157–84.
19. Milliman care guidelines. Available at https://www.mcg.com/content/about-mcg. Accessed 23 April 2016.
20. Mitus AJ. Birth of InterQual. Prof Case Manag. 2008;13(4):228–33.
21. Slee VN. Report of the conference on hospital discharge abstracts systems. Med Care. 1970;8(4 Supplement: Hospital Discharge Data):34–40.
22. Luft HS. The professional activity study of the Commission on Hospital and Professional Activities: a user's perspective. Health Serv Res. 1983;18(2):349–52.
23. Boucher A, Bowman S, Piselli C, Scichilone C (2010) The evolution of DRGs. J AHIMA web exclusive. Available at http://bok.ahima.org/doc?oid=106590#.Vz3ODjUrLRY. Accessed 23 April 2016.
24. National Healthcare Expense Tables. Available at https://www.cms.gov/research-statistics-data-and-systems/statistics-trends-and-reports/nationalhealthexpenddata/nhe-fact-sheet.html. Accessed 23 April 2016.
25. Burwell SA. Setting value-based payment goals—HHS efforts to improve U.S. Health Care. N Engl J Med. 2015;372:897–9. doi:10.1056/NEJMp1500445.
26. Coffey CE, Goodman RJ, Chang KM, Griner T, Dailey F, Nuckols TS. Implementing guideline-based indications for cardiac monitoring at Cedars-Sinai Medical Center. Abstract presented at the 2016 Society of Hospital Medicine Annual Meeting, San Diego, CA, 6–9 March 2016.
27. James B, Savitz LA. How intermountain trimmed health care costs through robust quality improvement efforts. Health Aff. 2011;30(6):1185–91. doi:10.1377/hlthaff.2011.0358.
28. Pronovost P, Needham D, Berenholtz S, Sinopoli D, Haitao C, Cosgrove S, Sexton B, Hyzy R, Welsh R, Roth G, Bander J, Kepros J, Goeschel C. An intervention to decrease catheter-related bloodstream infections in the ICU. N Engl J Med. 2006;355:2725–32. doi:10.1056/NEJMoa061115.

Chapter 5
Aligning Medical Staff Within the Academic Medical Center

Victoria G. Hines and Michael F. Rotondo

Introduction

The 1200 physicians of the University of Rochester Medical Faculty Group (URMFG) have a unique advantage in the turbulent health care environment; they are part of a large fully integrated medical center enterprise with a reputation for sound strategic evolution that understands the essential role that physicians play in redesigning the care system and assuring financial strength. But ongoing success will be heavily dependent on the organization's ability to continue to transform a loosely aligned medical staff into a value-driven multispecialty group practice that stimulates a thriving future for the practice, the overall health care system and the academic mission.

Historically, the medical staff at the University of Rochester Medical Center (URMC) has been closely aligned with their academic departments. It is, after all, a research university that attracts some of the best basic and translational scientists for whom great patient care is rivaled by world-renowned academic and creative work. In 1996, faculty practice visits totaled less than 500,000 annually, and the majority of those visits were in the service of resident clinics. Today, the faculty still supports approximately 500,000 resident-driven clinic visits, but also conducts an additional one million ambulatory visits for both fee-for-service and value-based insurance plans. The sheer size of the faculty practice has required a transformational change in focus and leadership; the practice is now far more dependent on patient care revenues to support research and educational missions; URMFG is now equally focused on recruiting and retaining great clinicians in addition to great scientists and similarly focused on access, quality, service, and cost.

V.G. Hines • M.F. Rotondo (✉)
University of Rochester Medical Faculty Group, University of Rochester Medical Center, 601 Elmwood Ave., Rochester, NY 14642, USA
e-mail: michael_rotondo@urmc.rochester.edu

© Springer International Publishing Switzerland 2017
H.C. Sax (ed.), *Measurement and Analysis in Transforming Healthcare Delivery*, DOI 10.1007/978-3-319-46222-6_5

This chapter focuses on the transformation of the URMFG practice from a federated academic model to a multispecialty group practice model. Now, 3 years into the transformation, the impact is already clear. Physicians are better informed about the business environment, more accountable for patient outcomes and practice efficiency, and poised for success in evolving payment models that include narrow networks and risk-bearing contracts. The maturation of the faculty group results from a shared vision and practice principles, a strong new governance structure, a focus on key performance metrics, and a compensation plan that rewards achievement on those metrics. That said, the critical feature of this latest chapter in the development of URMC has been a constant focus on the academic mission as well, a differentiating feature that defines our identify.

Creating a Shared Vision for the Future

In his book, *Reinventing American Health Care*, Ezekiel Emanuel noted that "physicians will be caught in a misalignment with an outdated business model" [1]. Evolving transparency in quality reporting and pricing means that physicians and other providers feel the pressure of increased accountability for value-based service delivery. The misalignment festers in the structural deficiencies in the system; fee-for-service payment models that encourage revenue growth through volume continue to live alongside new payment models that incentivize cost efficiency and quality outcomes. It is a difficult environment to navigate and strength will come from collective agreement and alignment on core values and principles that guide strategic decision-making.

One thing is clear, "alignment" of medical staffs and medical groups can occur in a whole host of models, each being unique to the culture of that particular group, as influenced by the local competitive health care environment as well as local laws and statutes. Overarching are the federal mandates of the Stark Laws that impose clear restrictions and guidelines referable to issues of anti-trust, anti-kickback, fair market value, and commercial reasonableness. These requirements influence the relationships between groups of physicians, hospitals and insurers, all of which must be carefully navigated to stay in a safe harbor and well within the bounds of the law. Many academic practices functioned in the past as a group of loosely affiliated federations that were legally separate and distinct from any and all definitive care facilities. However, this model does not promote cohesion and alignment amongst primary care physicians, specialists, and hospitals. Moreover, with the move to value-based payment across episodes of care which span ambulatory—acute inpatient and post acute phases, it becomes quite challenging to successfully negotiate contracts with payers given the complexity of the relationships. Moreover, private practice physician groups have coalesced into Independent Physician Associations (IPA) in an effort to leverage collective bargaining power with both hospitals and insurance entities. Some have utilized a "messenger model" such that an agent negotiates non-price-related stipulations in contracts with payers to avoid "price-fixing" while navigating the stormy waters of both gain and risk sharing arrangements.

Never has "alignment" been so important across health care entities as it is today in the current era of gain sharing on the way to full risk assumption. To succeed in risk share requires that all entities involved in either an individual episode of care or in the management of the overall care of a group of patients have clear visibility on predetermined benchmarks for performance, real-time clinical decision support and ongoing analysis, and identification of gaps in care. This is no small task and one at which health systems across the nation are working arduously to achieve at no small expense. Physician groups, advanced practice providers, hospitals, home care agencies, long-term care facilities, and virtually all other elements of the system will have to work together cohesively to meet the goal of providing high value care for patients in the future in hopes of succeeding in a full risk environment.

How can a change toward alignment of such a diverse group of elements in a rapidly changing and uncertain environment be engineered? The first key tenets of effective change management are to create a sense of urgency and then form a powerful coalition that creates and attains a vision for the future [2]. A sense of urgency can only come from a shared understanding of the challenges posed by health reform and the regional competitive environment, both of which either directly or indirectly pose a threat to the academic mission. Leaders should not assume that each faculty member is well aware of the broader impact of changes in payment strategies, particularly if their own professional revenue has not been affected. The transformation of the URMFG began with group and individual conversation about the declining financial health of the medical center, the pending declines in Medicare, Medicaid and commercial insurance reimbursement rates, and the increasingly competitive environment driven by patients and employers who seek easy access to great care. Specialists gained a better understanding of the unique challenges that their primary care partners faced in developing patient-centered medical homes and performing within the first accountable care contracts. Primary care providers learned to appreciate the taxing burden on specialists to change the way they provide care when their revenue is still largely based on volume-driven fee-for-service rates. A powerful coalition began to form naturally as key faculty leaders recognized that future success required a strong, high-performing multispecialty group practice.

Since its founding, the URMFG has been a loosely organized federation of 22 independent departments and 120 divisions, each operating with their own expectations for practice performance. Early on, leaders began to paint a picture of the future with images. "URMFG United" denoted a new sense of unity, and a clear image of the desired multispecialty model put the patient experience at the center (Fig. 5.1).

Most importantly, faculty practice leaders adopted a set of principles and values that would guide strategic and business decision-making. Those principles included the desire to deliver integrated, coordinated care and high-end, consistent customer service through a unified, consistent approach for the group practice. Faculty agreed that all decisions would be guided by department knowledge and successes as well as industry best practices as a means of honoring the existing expertise among colleagues. They agreed to consistently meet high levels of performance, with a focus on efficient processes and overall reduced cost per service. Finally, they underscored the need for transparency and committed to sharing successes and challenges and to recognizing the impact of change on staff and faculty.

URMFG *United*

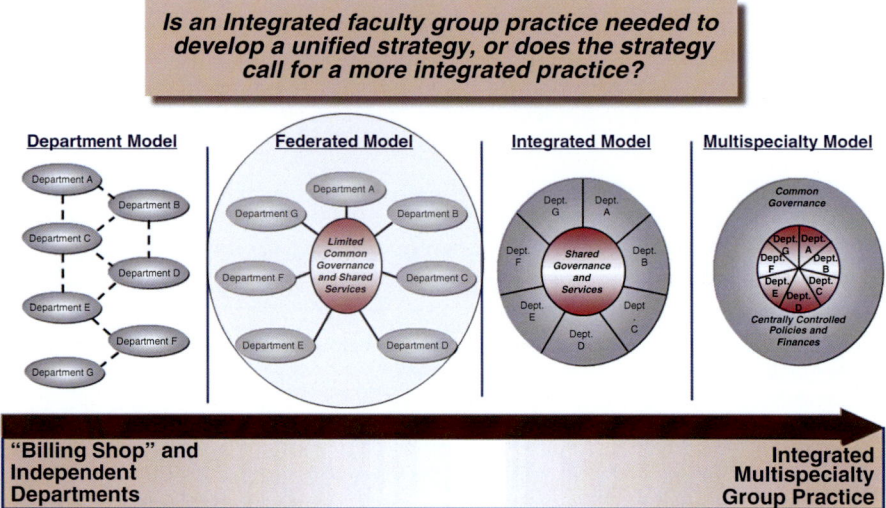

Fig. 5.1 Models in evolution to a fully integrated multispecialty group practice (Reproduced with permission from ECG Consulting Management—Boston, Massachusetts)

Transforming Governance: By the Faculty and for the Faculty

A strong and transparent governance structure, led by Department Chairs, has been the cornerstone of success in this movement. Today, Department chairs and more than 55 faculty members steer the direction of the group practice through a committee structure charged with making specific progress toward the vision of a thriving multispecialty practice. Each committee is active in meeting its charge, and their work is continuously communicated to faculty through an intranet site devoted to URMFG United and through routine communication from the group's CEO. The governance structure is represented below. It has formed a foundational structure for growth of practice leadership in responsibility, authority, and accountability (Fig. 5.2).

Metrics Drive Performance

Evidence of culture change began to emerge when the faculty governance structure adopted standards for performance and published key metrics for success. Both the Finance and Clinical Operations Committees each focused on key performance

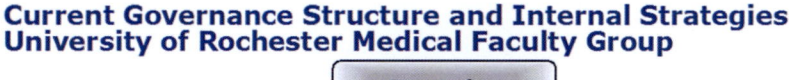

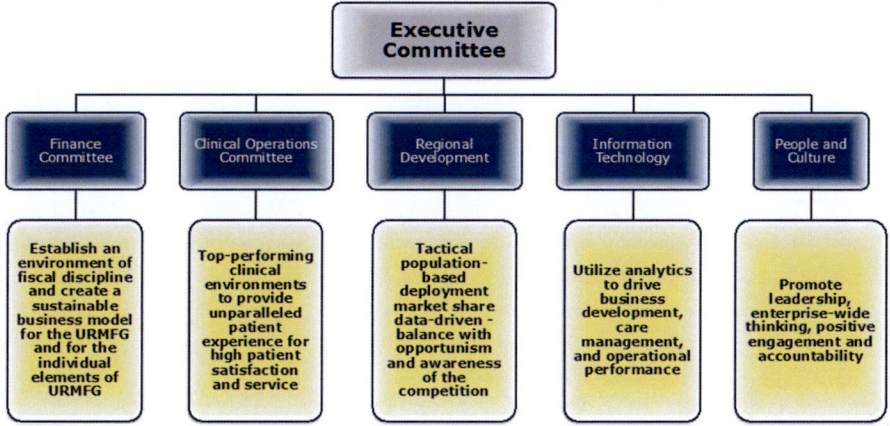

Fig. 5.2 Integrated Group Practice Governance: structure and function

indicators, developed measurement tools for those indicators, and communicated expectations widely and often to all faculty.

Key Performance Indicators

The Finance Committee routinely reviews individual department and overall URMFG financial performance and key benchmarks for efficient operations including: WRVUs per Faculty FTE; Encounters per Faculty FTE; Staff Salary Costs per Faculty FTE; and Total Expenses per Faculty FTE. Importantly, the committee established a rigorous process for the review of new business plans. Historically, individual divisions would expand business with a plan that was acceptable and affordable to the individual division. The faculty group therefore had little opportunity to grow business together or to take advantage of business efficiencies that come from expanding in multispecialty sites rather in a collection of individual offices. Moreover, expansion was only possible in departments that had enough cash on hand to fund acquisitions or new real estate. Today, practice expansions are typically multispecialty and the choice of location is more broadly influenced by competitive needs across departments and competitive forces in the market.

The Clinical Operations Committee focused on the practice metrics that would create access and value for patients. The committee benchmarked the practice behavior of other high-performing systems and developed 16 new policies that defined how URMFG practices would operate. Key performance standards included: 80 % of new patient visits would occur within 14 days of the visit request; fewer than 2 % of patient appointments would be "bumped" (rescheduled) by the practice;

patient encounters in e-record would be closed within 48 h; and specialists would communicate back to referring providers within 72 h.

Measurement Tools

Reflective of an aggressive revenue cycle culture, the practice had already developed a comprehensive performance dashboard for billing and revenue metrics. The use of that dashboard clearly supported performance excellence; URMFG ranks third across faculty practice plans for net collection efficiency [3].

New dashboards had to be developed to drive practice performance in delivering an excellent patient experience. An interactive tool was developed to track metrics for patient access, provider communication, and patient satisfaction at the department, division, and individual provider level (Fig. 5.3).

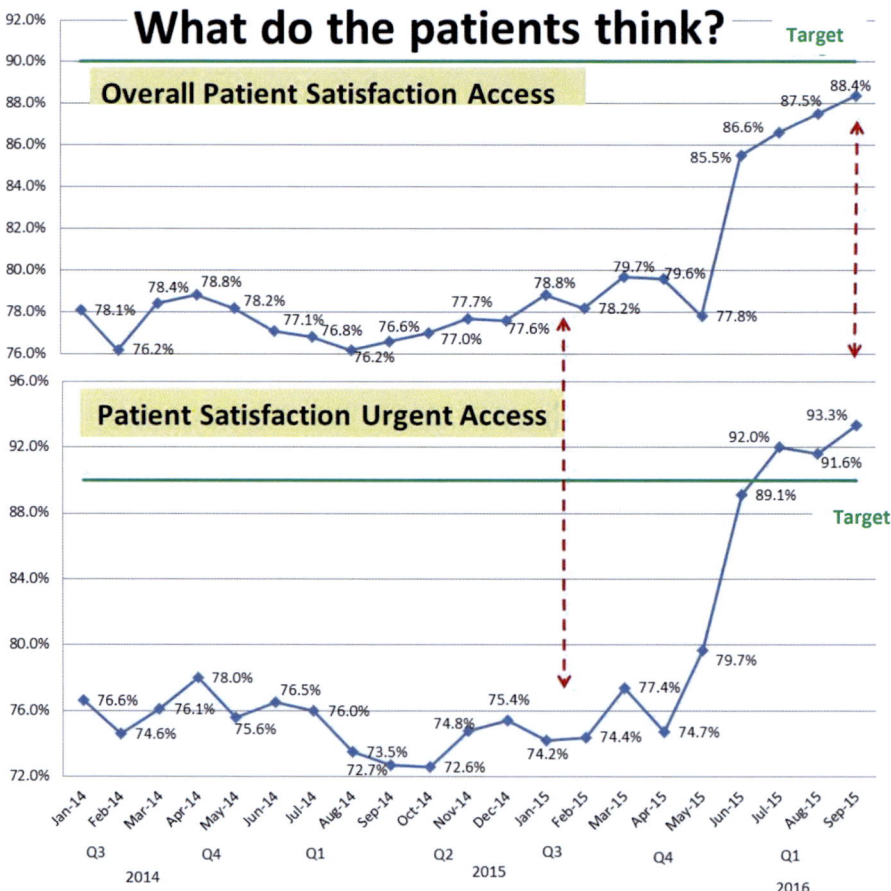

Fig. 5.3 Patient satisfaction monitoring

Year over Year Key Metrics Trends

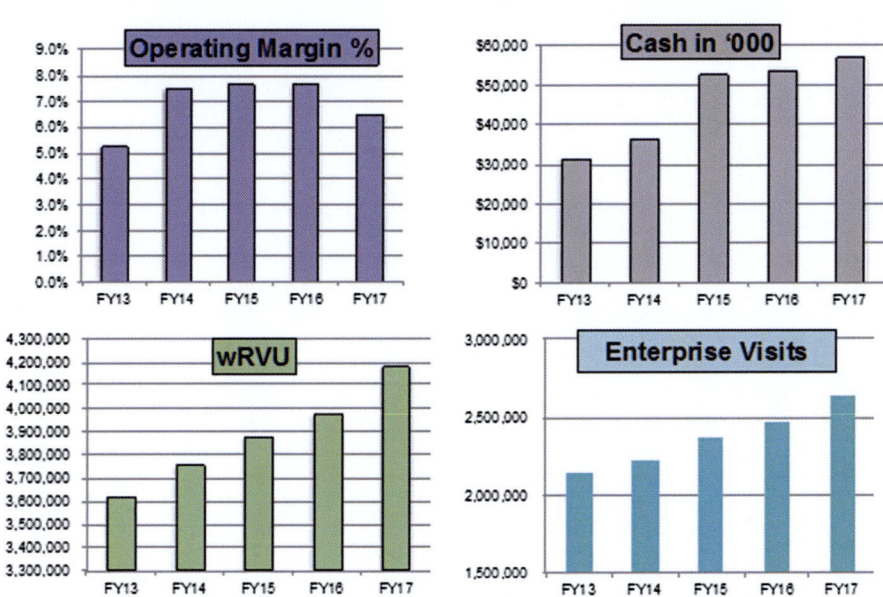

Fig. 5.4 Integrated group practice performance dashboard

Moreover, group practice dashboards were developed to emphasize performance of the entire multispecialty practice in an effort to highlight overall success (Fig. 5.4).

Communicating Performance

Use of these new metrics and a move to full transparency in performance benchmarking began with a "soft" launch; the first performance reports were published for the use of Chairs and their administrators only, and for the purpose of assuring that the data were reliable. As expected, the first 6–12 months of data sharing provoked concern over poor–fair performance against target metrics. Department Chairs and URMFG staff took deep dives into data integrity and identified department-specific opportunities to improve performance.

Performance reports were widely shared at department faculty meetings, at "town hall" style URMFG faculty meetings, and through written communication. For the last 12 months, departments have been accountable for continued improvement. That accountability is supported through routine meetings between department and URMFG leaders to identify trends and develop action plans for improvement. Overall, the URMFG governance structure and the Board of the medical center routinely review practice performance metrics.

Table 5.1 Balanced metric approach to patient access performance

URMFG Access Dashboard

Metric	Enterprise	Aug '15	Sep '15	Oct '15	Nov '15	Dec '15	Jan '16	6 Month Average	Change from Prior Year
1	Visit Volume	168,582	179,266	193,559	171,038	182,219	173,668	178,055	↑13.0%
2	New Patient Visits	23,741	24,877	26,182	23,109	24,034	24,618	24,427	↑10.0%
3	New Patient Visits/Total Visits (%)	14.1%	13.9%	13.5%	13.5%	13.2%	14.2%	13.7%	↘-0.4%
4	New Patient Visits in 14 Days	13,366	13,931	14,898	12,918	12,618	13,565	13,557	↗1.4%
5	Booked/Available Hours (%)	51.2%	50.8%	51.7%	51.9%	51.2%	50.3%	51.2%	↓-8.4%
6	Closed Encounters	144,762	147,414	154,117	134,955	141,136	131,987	142,395	↑2.6%
7	New Patient Visits in 14 Days (%)	●56.3%	●56.0%	●56.9%	●55.9%	●52.5%	●55.1%	●55.5%	↓-4.8%
8	Bumped Appts within 60 days (%)	○2.4%	○2.3%	○2.4%	○2.3%	○2.4%	●2.6%	○2.4%	→0.0%
9	CG CAHPS Appointment as Soon as Needed (%)	●96.3%	●96.0%	●95.7%	●96.7%	●96.8%	NA	●96.1%	↑17.8%
10	CG CAHPS Urgent Appointment as Needed (%)	●91.6%	●93.3%	●92.7%	●93.5%	●92.1%	NA	●92.5%	↑18.7%
11	CG CAHPS See Provider within 15 Minutes (%)	●85.6%	●87.4%	●86.5%	●88.2%	●86.7%	NA	●86.7%	↑4.2%

Importantly, the practice has already evolved its understanding of the value of each metric and has a more balanced view of success. For example, the initial focus for improved access to care was the ability to get all new patient visits scheduled within 14 days. However, the practice is currently unable to track how many patients are offered and decline visits within that 14-day period, and is now equally focused on improving access to urgent care and on meeting individual patient expectations regarding their access to care. This shift resulted in the development of both a more comprehensive understanding of "access to care" for patients and more sophisticated set of metrics to measure performance (Table 5.1).

Since the introduction of the dashboards in 2014, URMFG providers have accommodated over 200,000 additional patient visits annually with the same number of clinical faculty. At the same time, access to urgent care has increased dramatically, as has patient satisfaction with their access to care. Much of this success has come from the sharing of best practices across specialties; faculty are working together to assure that patients have the same remarkable experience with each provider they interact with.

Compensation That Rewards the Right Achievements

In tandem with the development of practice policies and new performance indicators, a Compensation Committee was tasked with establishing a master compensation plan that would support URMFGs new definitions of success. Chaired by a respected academic department chair and facilitated by an outside by ECG Consulting (A Boston-based health management consulting firm), the committee's work included faculty forums for input, review of external faculty practice plans, and modeling of various plan options. The final plan was adopted in 2016, and is based on assuring that faculty are compensated at market competitive rates.

The plan includes a philosophical shift in incentives for performance. Historically, faculty were generally compensated based on their own net revenue minus expenses associated with their individual practice. A few departments had begun to include performance metrics based on quality outcomes and academic performance, but there was no enterprise expectation to do so. The new plan includes expectations for achieving productivity benchmarks, and for meeting group objectives across all three missions. For Chairs and faculty alike, at least 20 % of annual compensation will now be tied to performance against department-specific objectives that could include improved access to care, achievement of contract-based quality metrics, achievement of selected team-based objectives, and meeting goals for both research and educational performance.

Plan development took longer than anticipated. Early and often, faculty expressed anxiety over the objectives of the plan and the change that it could mean to their income. Highly compensated specialists were concerned that some of "their" revenue would be used to fund faculty compensation in departments that generate less patient care revenue. Primary care providers were hopeful that the new focus on team-based and access outcomes would result in improved compensation for work they had already been committed to but not compensated for. URMFG leadership and the Compensation Committee spent several months engaging faculty in individual and specialty-specific discussion to answer questions and to listen to input that helped to shape the final plan. The key to success in this phase of development was aggressive faculty engagement and reliance on the governance structure to make the tough decisions.

As national benchmarks were reviewed, it became clear that there was significant misalignment between faculty productivity and their related compensation. In general, URMFG faculty had considerably higher clinical productivity and lower salaries than their peers at other institutions. That fact was used in two ways to further align and engage faculty in considering themselves part of high-performing group practice. First, both URMC and URMFG leadership publicly noted the success and commitment of faculty in achieving group and medical center objectives and in contributing to improved access and excellence in clinical care. Transparent review of productivity and salary benchmarks occurred in faculty meetings, in URMFG governance meetings, in Medical Center leadership meetings and at Board meetings. Medical Center leadership and individual faculty members have now begun to reshape their view of the practice; they better recognize the value and hard work of the faculty in achieving enterprise-wide success. Second, the URMFG CEO committed to narrowing the gap between pay and productivity by infusing new dollars to support the faculty group. Those dollars will be sourced from business improvement plans, aggressive value-based rate negotiations, and more efficient service delivery approaches. The new compensation plan will therefore start from a position of strength; a majority of faculty will see an increase in their base pay to assure that their compensation reflects their already high productivity. Most importantly, faculty governance will be held accountable for the proper implementation, ongoing execution, and compliance with the master compensation plan.

Cultural Challenges

It will take several years to fully accomplish the cultural shift that aligns the medical staff around shared objectives of the medical center relative to excellence in clinical care and exemplary research and education in the paradigm of the new health care environment. Some culture change is already evident. The governance structure has clearly evolved, with faculty making decisions based on what is best for the group and the enterprise rather than for individual departments. The most notable example is in the Finance and Executive Committees' decision to use specialty-designated incentive dollars derived from a gain share contract to support the group's safety net primary care practices and advance the global objectives of the clinically integrated network. URMFG leaders recognized that decision as demonstration that their thinking had changed and that they are both empowered to and capable of acting like a group practice on behalf of the overall organization.

Other evidence of culture change is in the nature of daily dialog among faculty and their leaders. Two years ago, angst and anger was prevalent as faculty sought to understand the purpose and value of the group's transformation. They questioned the integrity of all data and reports. They expressed concern over fears of lost compensation and lost control over their daily practice. And they noted the failures of their colleagues in meeting performance metrics as a way of justifying their own performance. Today, discussion focuses on finding best practices among their colleagues and on working together on new growth initiatives. There is less concern over loss of individual department autonomy and more focus on the responsibility of individual faculty members and departments in contributing to the success of the whole. While academic recruits remain essential, chairs and chiefs are focused on recruiting excellent clinicians who can help achieve patient access and patient experience metrics.

Maintaining Medical Staff Alignment

Despite the transformation in culture, faculty turnover has been minimal. Throughout this time, there has been active acknowledgement that faculty recruitment and retention is largely dependent on the *physician* experience. Working conditions and compensation are of utmost importance. It is no secret that a fully engaged, healthy workforce is key to meeting any performance expectations. A constantly changing reimbursement environment, pressure to perform in a value-driven health system, the challenges inherent in the use of electronic record systems, and known work-life balance issues are perhaps the biggest threat to the success of academic medical centers today. Further faculty alignment with shared values requires that the practice now use its strong governance structure to explore and invest in technology and processes that improve daily workflows and hence work life. Faculty will feel supported and capable of achieving performance targets when colleagues responsible for the "systems" of care work collaboratively with them in improving those systems.

Some of this work has already begun. URMFG supports a Center for Clinical Innovation tasked with identifying technological options to improve physician workflows. The Center has already developed and implemented biometric authentication for electronic record access and a streamlined approach to complying with state laws related to prescription monitoring of controlled substances. The innovation team is now focused on reducing physician burden in use of the new electronic revenue cycle system.

URMFG also supports a physician wellness program. In its infancy, the program is intended to keep the temperature of faculty satisfaction and to develop solutions to common dissatisfiers. Additionally, it provides support to individual faculty members who need assistance with mental health and wellness.

For the foreseeable future, URMFG leadership will have to find the balance between supporting strong culture change through a focus on accountability for established performance metrics with sensitivity to faculty well-being. Medical staff have and will continue to align around a system of shared values if they feel well represented and governed, well compensated, and respected by their colleagues across the health system.

References

1. Emanuel EJ. Reinventing American health care: how the affordable care act will improve our terribly complex, blatantly unjust, outrageously expensive, grossly inefficient, error prone system. New York: Public Affairs; 2014. p. 268.
2. Kotter J. Leading change: why transformation efforts fail. Harvard Business Review Best of HBR; 2007. p. 1–10.
3. Vizient, Inc. Faculty Practice Solutions Center FY15 billing office survey. 2015.

Chapter 6
Aligning Healthcare Systems

Thomas R. Graf and Glenn D. Steele Jr.

Introduction

Geisinger Health System (Geisinger) is an integrated health services organization widely recognized for its innovative use of the electronic health record and the development of care delivery models such as ProvenHealth Navigator® and ProvenCare®. As one of the nation's largest health service organizations, Geisinger serves more than three million residents throughout 45 counties in central, south-central, and northeast Pennsylvania, and also in southern New Jersey with the addition of AtlantiCare, a National Malcolm Baldrige Award recipient. The physician-led system comprises approximately 30,000 employees, including nearly 1600 employed physicians, 12 hospital campuses, two research centers, and a 510,000-member health plan, all of which leverage an estimated $8.9 billion positive impact on the Pennsylvania economy. Geisinger has repeatedly garnered national accolades for integration, quality, and service. In addition to fulfilling its patient-care mission, Geisinger has a long-standing commitment to medical education, research, and community service. But more importantly, Geisinger has served as a national model for innovation not only in the reliable delivery of measurably better care, but also in partnering with private physicians, hospitals, and post-acute providers to deliver that care across the communities we serve. *While Geisinger is a prototypical integrated delivery system, it is not a closed shop.* In 2015, only about 30 % of the patients that saw a Geisinger physician or hospital carried Geisinger Health Plan (GHP) insurance, the remaining 70 % the traditional mix of Medicare, Medicaid, and multiple commercial insurers both national and regional. Similarly,

T.R. Graf, M.D. (✉)
The Chartis Group, 108 Oak Lane, Pine Grove, PA 17963, USA
e-mail: thomasgraf@comcast.net

G.D. Steele Jr., M.D., Ph.D.
xG Health Solutions, 100 N. Academy Ave., MC 22-01, Danville, PA 17822, USA

© Springer International Publishing Switzerland 2017
H.C. Sax (ed.), *Measurement and Analysis in Transforming Healthcare Delivery*, DOI 10.1007/978-3-319-46222-6_6

of the half million members of GHP, only about 30 % receive their care from a Geisinger-employed physician or Geisinger-owned hospital. The remainder gets their care from the 30,000 private physicians and over 100 private hospitals that are part of the network. Developing the capability to support, influence, and re-engineer the care delivered across this span required vision, disciplined process and relationship development, data aggregation and dissemination, innovative solutions and tools. Most importantly, perhaps, was having energized and committed physician and administrative leaders who could transform that data into information that was understandable and actionable by medical professionals, and who know what to do to achieve a different outcome. It required the various elements of the integrated systems to coordinate their interactions and meet the reasonable expectations of committed partners with high-reliability over many years to achieve sustained improvement. It required continuous adaption as market changes continued to accelerate. Finally, it demanded constant vigilance to prevent errors in leadership, planning, execution, and adaptation. In the end, we had transformed our internal culture to one of the team care, data, high reliability, and innovation, and then shared elements of that with our partners.

This chapter will focus on the journey to create the performance, reliability, and partnership expertise that enabled that reputation. Starting in 2004, after the near-death experience of a failed 2000–2001 merger with Penn State Hershey, a dramatic change was required to reinvigorate a clinic model health system. The first several years were devoted to stopping the loss of money, time, and talent and to creating a stable base from which to grow an academically powered, population health-focused enterprise that, with the private practice and community partners, would improve the health status of the people of central Pennsylvania. The internal cohesion and external alignment that powered the transformation of care delivery was formed around a common vision for better care for every patient, every time.

Creating a Shared Vision for a System and Its Partners

In the 1990s, healthcare reform centered on the idea of high quality versus low cost, and there really was no debate with everyone interested in high quality and assuming that this meant high cost by default. By 2000 though, evidence showed that not only was quality versus cost best seen as a scatter gram but emerging data indicated that a correlation between cost and quality existed and that, in fact, higher quality was associated, often, with lower cost. While this was revolutionary for medicine, it is hardly novel for other, more mature industries. Also, while the quality of the medical evidence continued to increase, the likelihood that any given patient would receive all the care they should, and nothing extra, was basically a coin flip as shown by the seminal New England Journal of Medicine article in 2003 [1]. Meanwhile the drive for transparency of cost, quality, and operational data continued to grow. These forces combined to create the need for a new health system. One focused on improving quality to reduce total cost of care and doing so by innovating new ways to deliver all the necessary care and only that care, as well as the need to move the patient/family from a sometimes unwillingly passive recipient of care to an active team member with roles and responsibilities. The other emerging drive was the need for patient/provider/payer partnerships, soon to be joined by employer and public/private partnerships to actually create a sustainable model to allow for the optimal health status for all people. These partnerships need also to underline the fact that in order to truly impact healthcare, information and care innovation cannot remain isolated within an organization.

These elements were interwoven to create the vision for the second 5 years in which all members of Geisinger crafted: quality, innovation, expanding the clinical market, and securing the legacy, as the strategic differentiators that would lead to better healthcare for all. They also served to align the various elements both within and outside of the health system—Geisinger physicians, private physicians, Geisinger Health Plan, Geisinger and private hospitals, Geisinger and private post-acute elements, and patients.

For quality and innovation, which were tightly linked, we set out to define rigorously and granularly what the best practice was, not for isolated elements, but for whole episodes of care or for comprehensive condition management from the patient-centered perspective of what would actually improve health. We then set about designing ways to reliably deliver that care, doing so, and proving the impact with hard end-points as the means to both improve health locally, but also to impact health delivery regionally and nationally. Ultimately, both in system (vertical integration) and out of system (horizontal integration) were leveraged.

The expanding the clinical market element was focused on two main goals. The first was on the traditional expansion of the service area, but the second was on driving care closer to the patient. This involved partnering with various local physician groups and hospitals in a very market-specific manner. We worked with a dozen private hospitals, some of which had embedded adult and pediatric hospitalist programs, in communities where we had an ambulatory presence and thousands of private physicians, primary care, and subspecialty based, for other care. The idea in each market was the care that could be done well and safely locally, should be as it was best for the patient and often lower cost than our quaternary and tertiary centers. What we needed to do, however, was to improve the quality, outcomes, and reliability of that care. It also resulted in various virtual care and convenient care applications and expanding the capabilities of the patient portal to integrate patient-entered data and engaging in shared decision-making in a robust sense.

Finally, the securing of the legacy differentiator was designed to ensure the sustainability of the innovations by improving the care delivery experience and developing the people expected to deliver that better care. By focusing time and effort on improving the ability of medical professionals to deliver better care, the waste, as well as the frustration level, in the system was reduced. This, in turn, allowed better focus and streamlined improvements in the quality and service of the care provided to the patients and families. Particular attention was applied to developing competent and committed physician leaders. Physicians who are fully engaged can drive, disproportionately, the results in quality, cost, and service. They are harder to find or create than excellent administrative leaders, who are obviously also critical to this process. Emerging leaders were identified early, given both didactic and experiential learning opportunities, and mentored in ever expanding real operational roles. They needed both the background skills and serial real-world experiences to truly lead other physicians in the challenging transitions. Considerable effort was made to ensure that they were ready for this challenge.

Together these elements created both a sustainable difference in the market and, more importantly, served as a unifying platform. This vision for patient-centric, reliably better health at lower cost, delivered closer to the patient via a system focused on improving the experience of medical professionals in so doing, served as a rallying point internally and an effective leverage point for nascent partnerships.

Harnessing Clinical Redesign to Hard-Wire the Alignment Performance

Once the "hearts and minds" are engaged in order to produce reliable and sustainable improvement, the entire system of care needs to be redesigned and the improvements designed built into the new, but soon to be standard, process of care. We strongly embraced Don Berwick's "All-or-None" philosophy of performance measurement for all elements of best care [2]. Meaning if there were nine specific elements to optimal care of a chronic disease, we looked, from a patient perspective, at whether or not they received all elements of care, and nothing extra. If they did receive all the care they should, they counted in the numerator and the denominator. If they missed even one element, they were only in the denominator. Thus, we measured how many of the people we cared for with a certain condition received all the care we had agreed was important. Setting the bar exceptionally high drove the system to understand the fundamental need for change. It was very clear to the doctors, nurses, and other medical professionals that remembering better and working harder was not going to ensure optimal care. There is no way to remember better such that hundreds of open heart patients would receive all 42 elements of best care for coronary artery bypass graft surgery starting with the surgical evaluation and ending with the return on the patient to usual care or ensure that the 20,000 patients with diabetes had all nine intermediate outcome and process measures deemed critical to their optimal care completed. Developing a system that ensured that the care was physician/patient dyad directed and team delivered was critical. By understanding the optimal role of each team member, redesigning the people workflows, and then creating electronic accelerators to reduce the "friction" of providing the best care and enhance the reliability, we were able to stop relying on the heroic efforts of diligent individuals to produce great results. By turning the process of care delivery around and starting with the goals from a patient perspective, we created an aspirational vision that demanded both better quality and better patient and professional experience [3] which, in turn, led to lower cost [4] and a more sustainable system. These innovations were again offered to aligned partners to enhance their performance and increase their engagement. Geisinger Health Plan developed a web portal version of these improvements, metrics, measures, targets, and feedback and shared it with the private practices with whom they worked. They also supported the individual practices redesign efforts in order to enhance performance and included people and technology systems built to improve reliability. Similarly, the Keystone Accountable Care Organization worked with the members to re-engineer their work flows and electronics to translate the innovations into highly reliable but group-specific programs based on the same principles and design but adapted to their unique environment. These innovations resulted in significant performance improvement and connected each element more tightly to the organization but, most importantly, the shared work and success created the people connections necessary to enable true synergy and trust-based relationships for long-term joint success.

Creating the Capacity to Reliably Innovate

In order to move beyond a single, if important, innovation and truly leverage it as an alignment strategy, we needed to create a disciplined process to continually and persistently innovate and improve—an innovation engine—to align the health system. It serves two needs—the need to develop mastery and the need to be part of a winning team and have some measure of control over one's own destiny, particularly in the face of the dramatic and unsettling changes in healthcare finance and delivery. This innovation engine needs to be the focus of significant leadership time and commitment. Senior leaders need to participate and resource a group that is focused on key clinical and operational challenges and tasked with designing new responses to them. Obviously, support for local level, often evolutionary rather than revolutionary ideas, also has to be present, but it is not a substitute for focused central effort. Once the ideas are generated and a prototype solution developed, a small best practice team with care redesign, operations, analytics, and IT skill is tasked with developing the new people workflows and the electronic accelerators to ensure high reliability, simplified behaviors, and real improvement. Once this is tested in real-world settings, the group then deploys it across the network, and only after it is fully deployed and debugged, it is transferred to operations. This team creates a significant boost to the alignment of systems because it ensures that there is one standard approach, which is efficient and effective, used universally. This process is also very helpful in aligning elements outside of the system. The innovation itself is usually highly applicable and highly valuable to the outside physicians or facilities, but needs to be carefully adapted before it can be used in those settings. The best practice team can serve as consultants and supports for the private groups as they modify and adopt the innovation. Creating a purposeful team and process to reliably design, test, pilot, troubleshoot, and spread the innovation is an exceptionally important support for reliably innovating. Through this framework, additional systems of care covering other chronic diseases, as well as prevention, were created, deployed, and reliably and measurably improved outcomes. Additionally, the model was extended to include post-acute and specialty care–primary care connectivity.

The Role of Data, Metrics, and Analytics

The role of actionable information in the successful alignment of high performing healthcare organizations cannot be understated. The difficulty in translating the vast amounts of raw data into information, correlating that information to create real meaning, understanding the implications, knowing what to do to create a meaningful difference, and then reliably executing those changes to achieve that difference is an incredibly complex task. Only slightly less daunting is the need to focus on only those metrics that are critical to the broad success of the organization and develop an effective cascading function so that the local work elements, e.g., those actually directly supporting patients, can influence the metrics they are measured against. It is also critical to understand and agree how these both correlate with those system-level goals and meaningfully contribute to the health of the people for whom we are privileged to help.

Determining the system level goals is the first essential element. These need to be focused on long-term outcomes but impacted by the system in a realistic manner and timeline. They need to be broad enough to encompass the totality of the vision of the system and clearly translatable by the various divisions so as to be relevant to their constituents. They must be focused enough in number so as not to overly stretch available resources and generally derived from the strategic differentiators and seen as reliable and accurate proxies for performance. They also need to be seen as tied to meaningful outcome differences. So, the metric should be clearly tied to the strategy, represent actual performance, and be generally recognized that a change will result in a real difference in performance of the organization and/or improvement in the health of individuals and communities. From these metrics, the individual units then derive their specific metrics that are relevant to their populations and people. This process continues until we arrive at those units directly touching patients or directly supporting those that do. As an example, one Geisinger metric was observed to expected (O:E) mortality for the system. Each service line, each hospital, the health plan, etc. all developed metrics that were directly connected to this, and further, each unit created metrics that tied to the service line or facility goal in a direct fashion. So system O:E mortality was translated into service line and then specific procedural O:E ratios or specific hospital unit, say the surgical ICU O:E mortality ratio. With these specific metrics in place, then targets could be developed and specific tactics generated to drive improvement.

This metric also embodies the need to measure both internal performance (e.g., observed—our month—over-month results) compared to an external to the organization benchmark (e.g., expected—the industry standard in this case). The need to have an external comparator is critical as it gives relevance to performance and helps to reduce complacency. It also supports realistic targets and validates the importance of the metric, given that others have agreed it is important. Certainly, there will be some metrics that are important to an organization that do not have a readily available external benchmark, but the advantages of those that do are significant.

Setting realistic and achievable targets is the next step. Clearly driving maximal sustainable improvement in each metric is important but this must be balanced with achieving optimal performance across all domains. Leveraging external benchmarks and, where available, best in class local performance can assist with this. Target setting that is achievable by a meaningful subset of the units is critical to continued engagement of the teams. Geisinger generally used two to three levels of achievement for all metrics and targeted the lower performance metric so that 65–75 % of the work units achieved it, while setting the upper performance metric so that perhaps 25–35 % achieved it.

Reporting performance in a reliable and effective manner is an important factor as well. Reports need to be frequent enough that the impact of change, or lack thereof, can be recognized. They need to be presented in a fashion that is understandable and actionable and shows internal and benchmark performance simultaneously. For example, our diabetes bundled performance reports were generated monthly with composite and individual metrics shown with current, prior, and best-in-class performance achievement. Additional information such as specific tips to accelerate performance in lagging metrics were included so that work units could immediately consider options and move to action. The optimal frequency and format needs to be based on the metric and timeline to achieve real change.

Ideally, a team would be focused on managing performance on each of the major metrics and organized at a local, regional, and system-wide level. The various levels would have very different approaches to optimizing performance. Local teams would focus on those elements where local performance lagged overall performance, or elements of particular relevance or interest locally. Regional teams would determine the best means to optimize performance either through care system redesign or changes to the composition of the team or create electronic or other accelerators. The system-level team assesses the impact of the local and regional team and manages the overall delegation of resources. They also need to balance the performance across the various metrics. These teams ideally should be led by clinician leaders who can take all types of data, quality, cost, utilization, and operations; translate it into information that is understandable to broad clinical and nonclinical audiences; and also understand what changes are required in their work units to achieve a meaningful result. This skill set is important and needs to be carefully cultivated as it is one of the most critical steps.

The final piece, and one many organizations overlook, is to create a highly reliable process to deliver the improvements that were designed and piloted and to do so broadly across the network. This "hard-wiring" ensures both the cementing of the improvement and allows for the next wave of improvement to move ahead.

As we consider connecting data, metrics, and performance with physicians and facilities outside of the organization, several adjustments need to be made. First, while the organizational metrics and targets can serve as a template, adjustments will need to be made to ensure they are effective in the new environment and truly "owned" by the partners. Additionally, the data systems and reporting abilities will be different. Only by allowing the partners to jointly create the metrics, targets, and reporting will their full engagement be achieved. Often, as available, the organizational performance data can be shared but in a carefully considered manner so as not to antagonize, nor overwhelm, the partners, but instead to foster competition. Including some metrics where the partners have excellent and, perhaps, superior performance is often helpful to this end. This is not about "selling" the already predetermined metrics to the partners or creating "buy-in;" rather it is co-generating meaningful, measurable, and important measures for all in the partnership [5].

Finally, "Big Data" is a readily used and loosely defined term in healthcare. Like many of the emerging ideas of the past, it has been seen as the magic bullet for healthcare's woes. Certainly, there is an ever increasing stream of information about health-related activities, i.e., exercise data, calorie consumption, sleeping habits, and mental state that is streaming from complex wearable devices, and these are beginning to be incorporated into the medical records in some fashion. It is certainly likely that the ability to connect these data streams into the healthcare delivery system will provide incremental benefit, both to individuals, but more likely to whole populations. However, as we have seen, the difficulty in translating data into directly actionable information and then reliably leveraging that to help create improved health, is real, and we currently do not do this well for the typical medical data, "little data" and so prematurely adding additional complexity will not really add value. Understanding these new elements will be important only after a system has mastered the art of turning data into meaningful health improvements and thus can target interventions and nuance goals, based on patient preferences and behaviors using the new information.

Physician Leadership and Management

Creating truly aligned, engaged, and most importantly, committed physicians is arguably the most critical element both within and around health systems. While the above discussion will enable the potential for true commitment, the process is best ensured by having competent and driven physician leaders with superior administrative capacity. While these should be supported by able professional administrative colleagues, physician leaders are best able to have the tough conversations that enable shared accountability for performance, best able to sort through the real issues from less important, and the best able to translate organizational and physician perspectives and align them. They also understand both the clinical imperatives and organizational and administrative realties and where, how, and when to adjust, interpret, and insist. Physician leaders need both didactic skill development and opportunities for practical applications for them to build competence. We developed a program designed to identify and cultivate emerging physician leaders across multiple dimensions: operations, quality, innovation, and EMR optimization. A dedicated didactic program addressing typical operational issues focused on small spans of control and progressing as skills were created. Importantly, the real possibility of failure, with limited organizational and individual consequences, is important to develop real-world skills. Active mentorship to guide and shape the emerging leader, and shape the process as well is critical to the success of the program and the organization. The ability of leaders to both select and change development tracks, and to have exposure to multiple areas, as well as mentors, is helpful. These developing leaders can be excellent ambassadors and connections across the system and with the other community elements. They often are closer and have more time to commit to the outside connectivity, and this should be taken advantage of as relationships mature. Because they have typically gone through many of the changes and know what the adaptations require, as well as the fact that they are known to the outside partners, they often carry a very real credibility and can support the alignment by helping to translate and troubleshoot the innovation as it is adapted to the new environments. They often have more time to commit to the relationship and can, thereby, directly share in the work to transform. This shared leadership development and work often does more to further external trust and alignment than most programs.

The Special Case of Compensation

Much has been written about the role of compensation and funds flow in driving alignment and performance, and clearly it is not unimportant; however, compensation as a leverage point was used somewhat differently at Geisinger. Beth McGlynn's pivotal study over a decade ago highlighting the fact that just over half of all needed care was actually delivered to the patient, irrespective of whether it is preventive care, acute illness care, or chronic disease care, only points out part of the issue. The other piece was the corollary estimate that it would take 22 h per day for the average primary care physician to deliver all of the needed services. Clearly, you cannot pay anyone enough to maintain that pace. Additionally, commercial insurance companies for years have tried using pay for performance to improve something as simple as isolated HEDIS metrics with dismal results. While one can temporarily improve these scores, as soon as the compensated measure change, (colon cancer screening moving to breast cancer screening,) the performance in the initial metric falls back to baseline while the new metric improves. In response, insurers tried endlessly adding to the list of measures which in turn led to provider burnout and revolt. So what is the most effective role for funds flow and compensation in creating alignment? Clearly, the current system is fraught with too many paradoxes to be effective. The most obvious is the current Fee for Service practice of paying physicians for each day of work in the hospital but paying the hospital a set fee based on diagnosis and wondering why they are not working more closely together. Another is the zero sum game between providers and payers such that for one to win the other must lose. Obviously, paying for volume and expecting value is not workable, but we have also seen that to create sustained value creation, paying for value and magically expecting sustained, high-value performance is also unrealistic. Nevertheless, the kernel of the solution was uncovered by the pay for performance focus—it is the use of compensation to focus the attention of the medical professionals and help induce the acceptance of the changes necessary. So redesign the care system, then focus the medical professionals' attention on and participation with, the new system of care, in order to deliver sustained, high-value results. Additionally, there are corollary drivers of performance and alignment that can then be used. The most obvious of which is transparency of the performance data first of the individual, then the group, then across the enterprise, and finally publicly. This transparency is particularly effective with doctors and nurses as they are accustomed to excelling and are typically highly competitive with their peers. Coupling this with the sharing of best practices and support to make changes drives significant convergence of performance toward the high end of the curve. To be maximally effective, however, the newly transparent metrics need to be heavily influenced (not necessarily controlled) by the physician, accurately measured, indicative of medically important status, and comprehensive. They must also be easily measured, reported, and understood. Finally, as we discussed, the role of clinical leadership across all dimensions of performance, i.e., quality, cost, utilization, operations, and experience is key.

Aligning payers and providers relative to funds flow is more complicated. Shared savings was an early attempt at removing the barrier to joint success and can be highly effective in situations where significant opportunity exists for actual savings to be shared. Inevitably, however, these programs are subject to diminishing returns as the target is downwardly adjusted based on past performance improvements. Additionally, as "average" costs are used, there will be winners and losers amongst the providers. Especially in two-sided risk models, the payer is often held harmless, which does not necessarily promote optimal teamwork. For example, the CMS MIPS program essentially takes the cost of paying for superior performance out of the payments provided to those with inferior performance. This does not create the optimal environment for joint success, not that this is the goal of the MIPS program—which is designed to promote quality improvement and control cost for CMS. Ultimately, some form of risk-adjusted population payment where the healthcare providers assume risk for performance against a reference cost and insurers assume risk for true insurance issues (i.e., the prevalence of trauma in a population) with joint sharing of the gains and losses may provide the basis for true shared risk and reward.

Vigilance for the Four Modes of Failure: Leadership, Planning, Execution, Adaptation

Constant vigilance is required to maintain the alignment edge created by the previous disciplines. Failure comes in one of four guises, failure of leadership, failure of planning, failure of execution, and most often, failure of adaptation. Failures of leadership are often created when leaders focus too much on the skill set that historically worked without understanding how changes in technology, environment, or situation have materially altered the situation and will require a wholly new approach or leaders that have been promoted past their level of competence. High performing organizations typically avoid this failure. However, frequent leadership changes, particular in outward facing roles that interact with the eternal partners, can reduce the alignment as these are often relationship based on an individual, as well as organizational level.

Failures of planning are also rarely seen by competent organizations. If anything, they fall prey to excessive preparation and prolong the planning phase which can minimize the impact of the new strategy once finally implemented. Alignment requires often swift and focused execution and physicians, in particular, are concerned about prevarication. There is no such thing as the perfect plan, and in any case, all plans require adjustment based on the actual performance, rather than detailed projections and assumptions. Often, movement to rapidly implement and effectively iterate a "good" plan is far more effective than endlessly waiting to create the "perfect" plan. This is certainly true for organizations that have mastered rapid cycle adaptation and critical in the work of aligning external physicians and smaller, more nimble organizations.

Failure of execution, however, is all too common. Typically, the opportunity for this is created by establishing competing demands, goals, or priorities, or most often, by stretching resources beyond any manageable set of expectations. Expecting even a high performing organization to accomplish a large number of "top priority" goals is the surest recipe for disaster. This also then serves to demoralize the once high performing team, leading to further failures, defections, and ultimately the demise of the organization. Lack of appropriate resources, lack of appropriate performance measurement and feedback, or the lack of appropriate accountability can also lead to execution failures. Clear goals, adequate support, and direct measures with rapid cycle feedback to a clearly delineated leader is needed for success and will always lead to better alignment internally and externally. It will also establish an effective base to the relationship and allow for more complex and nuanced alignment and shared success going forward. Our ProvenHealth Navigator® Program illustrates this well. A single individual from GHP and from the clinical enterprise were identified and teamed together. They were given shared goals and metrics for success. These were measured continuously and reported broadly monthly. Most importantly, they had adequate resources in people, technology, and funding to ensure they could operationalize the plans. As the two groups continued to work together and achieve success, each element became easier and the alignment more natural, effective, and persistent.

The most common and most serious challenge for both new and established high-performance and high alignment organizations is failure of adaptation. This is the harder to mitigate and the most challenging to recognize. The need to adapt is ubiquitous and the impact of adaptation can only be truly measured retrospectively. This emphasizes the need to have all elements of the system continuously measuring its performance against not just internal but external benchmarks and making small adjustments to ensure not just month-over-month improvement, but improvement versus an external standard as well. This encompasses the fact that medicine is not static and that the organizational environment is not static and that in response to your advances, changes will occur, assumptions will be found to be incorrect, or anticipated progress will not be achieved. How the individuals and, thereby, the organization overall responds is critical in this time of supercharged change. Creating a culture of innovation that pervades the organization is the most effective means to addressing this critical potential failure point. With a culture of innovation, the understanding that continuous small-scale improvements and adjustments are necessary is clear and the infrastructure to assess and adapt is in place. This also ensures that the needed feedback information is broadly transmitted throughout the organization so that when these small scale, local efforts are, in fact, not achieving enough adaptation, that the organization as a whole can direct central resources to the effort or, conversely, understand that this is not likely to be successful, and direct resources away from the failing innovation to other more prosperous lines, depending on the centrality of the challenge.

Success in the future healthcare environment will require systems to develop high levels of internal cohesive and external alignment. The ability to create that alignment both is fostered by and, in turn, fosters the ability to support, influence, and re-engineer the care delivered across the span of a health system. This includes employed and affiliated physicians, owned and private acute care hospitals, skilled nursing facilities, ambulatory surgical centers, rehabilitation centers, home health agencies, and others. It requires vision, disciplined process and relationship development, data aggregation and dissemination, innovative care solutions and tools, and most importantly, energized and committed physician and administrative leaders with the right tools and levers to both accelerate and sustain the improvements. The ability to move from vision to innovation to better operations will support the alignment of internal and external partners and further accelerate success.

References

1. McGlynn EA, Asch SM, Adams J, Keesey J, Hicks J, DeChristofaro A, Kerr EA. The quality of care delivered to adults in the United States. N Engl J Med. 2003;348:2635–45.
2. Nolan T, Berwick D. All-or-none measurement raises the bar on performance. J Am Med Assoc. 2006;295(10):1168–70.
3. Bloom FJ Jr., Yan X, Stewart W, Graf TR, Anderer T, Davis DE, Pierdon SB, Pitcavage J, Steele GD Jr. Primary care diabetes bundle management: 3-year outcomes for microvascular and macrovascular events. Am J Manag Care. 2014;20(6):175–82. http://www.ajmc.com/publications/issue/2014/2014-vol20-n6/Primary-Care-Diabetes-Bundle-Management-3-Year-Outcomes-for-Microvascular-and-Macrovascular-Events.
4. Maeng D, Yan X, Graf TR, Steele Jr GD. Value of primary care diabetes management: long-term cost impacts. Am J Manag Care. 2016;22:e88–94.
5. Graf TR, Bloom Jr FJ, Tomcavage J, Davis DE. Value based re-engineering: 21st century chronic care models. Prim Care. 2012;39(2):221–40. http://dx.doi.org/10.1016/j.pop.2012.03.001.

Chapter 7
Influencing with Integrity

Michael R. Williams and Steven R. Sosland

It's not hard to make decisions once you know what your values are.

Roy E. Disney [1]

Introduction

Integrity is the concept of being consistent in your behaviors, your core values, the methods used to reach goals, and your personal principles followed to achieve desired outcomes. It can also be defined as the antithesis of hypocrisy. In fact, integrity is a very powerful force to influence both individuals and groups of people. This power is best summed up by a quote from former United States Senator Alan K. Simpson, "If you have integrity, nothing else matters. If you don't have integrity, nothing else matters" [2]. So integrity is the single value that should be found in all people, but especially those people who serve others in roles requiring mutual trust. Effectively building trust throughout a practice or organization is dependent on the integrity of others. Trust is the dependency on the proven or unproven integrity of others. It is also the confidence in knowing that the leadership of any group has the best interests of the providers and the entire team as top priority in every decision they make [3]. Providers of healthcare are clearly in the group that must be trusted [4]. Patients and fellow providers come to depend upon the integrity of all providers and fellow providers in a group of providers. If all providers are expected to have integrity then integrity is an

M.R. Williams, D.O., M.D., M.B.A. (✉)
University of North Texas Health Science Center, 3500 Camp Bowie Blvd.,
Suite 850, Fort Worth, TX 76107, USA
e-mail: Michael.williams@unthsc.edu

S.R. Sosland, M.B.A., B.S.
Office of People Development, University of North Texas Health Science Center,
4455 Camp Bowie Blvd, Suite 114, PMB 141, Fort Worth, TX 76107, USA

© Springer International Publishing Switzerland 2017
H.C. Sax (ed.), *Measurement and Analysis in Transforming Healthcare Delivery*, DOI 10.1007/978-3-319-46222-6_7

Fig. 7.1 Drivers of
performance, Ann
Rhoades, People Ink, 2013

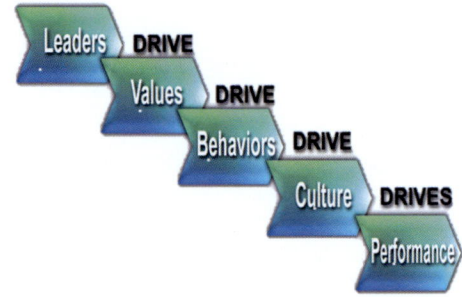

imperative for all provider group leaders. Leadership with integrity is an imperative for changing individuals and organizations to follow high-performing paths of achievement. This influential power can shape large and small cultures, guide directional change toward specific ends, create new leaders, and cause organizational alignment and engagement around a specific purpose and vision. This chapter discusses this specific power in the context of individual change, organizational change, and cultural transformation through the broader power of aligned core values. Provider groups often struggle with provider engagement and alignment. *Health systems have mistakenly believed that provider employment will yield provider engagement* [5]. *This is a false assumption.* When high-integrity provider leaders commit to aligning core values across a group of people, then following a set of defined specific behaviors for each of the core values, the power of cultural transformation begins. In fact, this values-based cultural transformation becomes a very important competitive differentiator for the organization as it leads directly to the creation of a high-performing metric-driven values-based organization. We know leaders drive values, values define behaviors, behaviors define the culture, and a values-based culture leads to high levels of performance [6]. It all starts with values-based, high integrity leadership (Fig. 7.1).

Influencing with Leadership

What is integrity and what does it mean for a leader to influence others with integrity? Let's begin with some definitions. Merriam-Webster gives three variations to the definition of integrity: incorruptibility, soundness, and completeness [7].

Integrity

The *incorruptibility* aspect of integrity refers to strict adherence to a moral code of values [8]. Soundness is described as an unimpaired condition [9]. Completeness is the quality or state of being complete or undivided [10]. Leading with integrity goes beyond a traditional definition of honesty or trustworthiness and combines all three of these aspects.

It is not enough to be honest. To be most effective, leaders must consistently adhere to a moral code of values shared by the team or organization they lead. It is not developed from the top down. It is developed by gaining an awareness of what values exist in the hearts of those in the organization and then identifying those commonly shared by all.

It is not enough to be trustworthy. Effective healthcare leaders build trust throughout the organization. This means having the courage and willingness to extend trust to others even before it is earned—to team members, other providers, and especially to patients. Through strict adherence to a common set of core values and building trust throughout the team, healthcare leaders can influence behavioral change and build a positive culture that leads to measurable changes in performance.

Leaders Drive Values That Drive the Organization's Culture

We need courageous leaders to transform the culture of healthcare from a provider-centric to a high-performing, patient-centric environment focused on creating value for patients. How do healthcare leaders transform our industry and achieve high-performing organizations? We believe it begins with a focus of leaders who drive values.

Merriam-Webster defines a person who leads as a guide or a conductor [11]. A guide is defined as a person who leads or directs other people on a journey, or a person who helps to direct another person's behavior, life, career, etc. [12]. A medical definition of conductor is defined as a bodily part (as a nerve fiber) that transmits excitation [13]. Combining these definitions and concepts we can develop the model of who we need in leadership positions to transform healthcare in America—a person who guides, leads, and excites a team or organization to begin a journey to establish a culture based on the common core values of the members of that group.

How does a leader of a small practice or a large hospital drive values throughout the organization? How do providers instill a culture of care throughout their practice? *Leaders drive values, not by creating a list for others to follow, but rather by creating an environment that allows each member of the organization to live their own values.* To create a values-based culture of care, leaders must understand their inability to give another adult values. Values are created during formative years by parents, grandparents, teachers, mentors, and those who influenced character development at a young age.

Leaders must listen to and collaborate with their team members to identify those common core values shared by all. These values serve as the moral compass on which the team can stay aligned during their journey. The leader's role is to model the values identified by the team and create the environment that allows the values to be lived every day. This all sounds like common sense and we agree it is. It is common sense, but it is not common practice. We need leaders unafraid to break the status quo. Only then can we truly transform the culture in the healthcare industry.

In a 2005 interview with Robert Galvin, Director of Global Health at General Electric, Don Berwick, founder of the Institute for Healthcare Improvement, saw the slow pace of improvement in U.S. healthcare as evidence of a failure of provider leadership. He concluded that external pressure would be necessary to move the system toward meaningful change [14].

In the interview originally published in *Heath Affairs*, Galvin asked, "Within those few [healthcare] organizations that have really taken on change, are you finding that they have what it takes to get that change done?" [14]

Berwick responded:

> ...the capability that is key to the proper allocation of resources and development of the proper workforce is leadership, and that's where we still lack traction. It's not that we don't have capable executives and committed boards. It's that the capable executives are still devoted to maintaining the status quo. And the hospital boards—I don't know if this should appear in print—but they're sort of out to lunch. They're good-hearted. They care about the organizations that they are stewards of; they respect the managers and the doctors. But they don't understand that they have a duty to cause change. And without executive and board leadership, I'm not sure we're going to get off the dime [14].

In an article published in the May/June 2008 issue of *Health Affairs*, Berwick, then President Obama's reported nominee to lead the Centers for Medicare and Medicaid Services, gave more details to the necessary pressure and laid out his vision for reforming the American healthcare system in what has come to be known as "The Triple Aim"—the simultaneous pursuit of three aims: improving the experience of care, improving the health of populations, and reducing per capita costs of healthcare [15].

Now, more than ever, we need courageous leaders to transform the culture of healthcare from a provider-centric to a high-performing, patient-centric environment focused on implementing Berwick's triple aim. Yes, we need courageous hospital administrators and board members willing to break away from the status quo. To effectively change our healthcare system it will take all involved, individual providers, and those in small groups. We need everyone to bring their values to work every day and help drive the behaviors that will change our healthcare culture.

Values Drive Behaviors

A behavior is defined as the response of an individual, group, or species to its environment [16]. A leader's greatest impact on determining the behaviors exhibited by the organization team members is to create the positive environment that allows individuals to live their values at work. The leader has the responsibility to model the group's desired behaviors.

In her book, *Built on Values*, Ann Rhoades describes how leaders drive the culture in their organizations. "When you are a leader of a company, division, or department, *every one of your actions matters, but particularly those that display your true values.* Your people talk about everything you do, and it becomes a part of your company's DNA. The best leaders understand the incredible impact their actions have on how employees behave every day" [17].

Creation of the Values-Based Culture

Many leaders and the organizations they lead pay far too little attention to the importance of understanding the specific culture they live and work in. The old adage is very true, every organization has a culture whether those in the organizations realize it or not. They give too little importance to the power of a culture to positively or negatively impact performance. As Peter Drucker once said "culture eats strategy for breakfast" [18]. The organization's culture is by far the most important single area for any leader's attention and focus. Culture is much more important than strategy, vision, or mission. In fact, many leaders mistakenly believe that a high-performing culture can be forced into existence by top-down actions and edicts. These same leaders struggle to understand how a high-performing culture truly comes into existence. We have learned that it only occurs through an intentional process of cultural transformation built upon aligned core values and a people first focus. Such a transformation will also require positive, optimistic, and committed leadership.

The first step is to determine if the organization or group of providers as a whole believes a new culture is needed. This will require a multifaceted assessment of the culture's current state. Is turnover high? How about provider satisfaction? How is the group doing on patient satisfaction? Are you losing "A" players and not dealing with the "C" players? Are you seeing only mediocre or average performance on the stated team goals and targets? Does the group have any stated values? If so, do the group members have any understanding or appreciation of these values and how to truly live them in their daily lives? Do the leaders set examples of living the group's core values via the specific behaviors? These are just a few of the questions the leaders of the group should be asking each other and the team in order to determine how much culture change is needed. *The reality is often that the group members know how broken the culture is far earlier than the leaders do.* Leaders need to be out among those on the "front line" to better understand how the culture is working and where it is not working in the best way.

Once the need for cultural change is determined, the second step is a continuation of the assessment process in order to begin listing the problems by specific categories. This begins to clarify the problems in specific categories. The areas of improvement in most group cultures revolve around a few key areas. For example, are there people problems like high turnover or poor recruitment? Any customer or patient satisfaction problems? How are the group quality scores? Any quality problems? What is the level of trust among the group members? How about the trust level of the group leaders? All of these questions must be addressed, in addition to many others, in order to build a robust plan for a high-performing culture transformation. So what current values are influencing the culture as it is? How can the leadership best summarize the findings of the values and culture assessment? Is there a need for values realignment and culture change based upon this summary? If so, is there a commitment from the group as a whole and the leadership to pursue a cultural transformation built upon newly aligned and identified core values?

These questions must be asked through the filter of the group's existing values in order to best understand how the cultural deficiencies are driven by meaningless values. The awareness of ineffective, meaningless values and a culture in need of overhaul should fuel the group's sense of urgency for new, aligned core values and a culture built on them. Meaningless values will lead to a meaningless culture. Well-developed and aligned core values with defined behaviors will drive the creation of a high-performing culture.

It is the careful construction of this "Values Blueprint" that will engage the frontline providers in the identification of the group's new values, align them, and build a plan to implement them into the very fabric of the group [19]. It becomes the foundational document from which everything else will come. Values, behaviors, cultural goals and expectations, problem areas of focus are all part of the blueprint. Then strategic initiatives, metrics, rewards and recognition programs, and communication strategies can all be developed. The group and its leaders should then begin building a systematic plan around the "Values Blueprint" to fully incorporate these values into the creation of the new culture. The new culture will drive new levels of group and individual performance.

High Performance as a Result of a Values-Based Culture

Once the "Values Blueprint" is completed and there is a strong commitment built to creating a new future for the group a high-performing culture can be created. Any successful high-performing culture starts with high-performing people and ends with high-performing people. The group has to commit to hiring "A" providers, those team members committed to living the group's values, and working every day to help the group achieve the defined goals. They are the frontline providers who show up every day looking for ways to add value to those they serve and their group. They are the ones the group strongly admires and values and they value their membership in the group. So you must hire "A" providers and work with "B" providers to improve and develop the skills needed to be "B+" providers or become "A" providers. "A" providers don't cause problems, add value, and improve almost every aspect of the group's performance. The "C" providers must be counseled and either must show significant improvement in a defined timeline or moved out of the group. Those providers who are not willing to work for the new culture live the new values or to assist in the new future becoming a reality should be given the opportunity and encouraged to find a new position elsewhere.

"A" and "B+" providers will want to know they are achieving the goals of the group and will want to be measured regularly. They want to be challenged! They also need to know they are appreciated for the value they add to the group and the group's patients and customers. Therefore, *values-based metrics need to be developed and a rewards and recognition program needs to be developed to incentivize the behaviors the group desires in the new culture.* With well-developed values-centered metrics and transparent reporting of results you will be creating a system of measuring and recognizing remarkable behavior and performance by team members. There should be at least two sets of metrics, one dashboard for the group performance and one for each individual team of providers who perform similar duties. Each dashboard should only have five to seven metrics and they should each directly relate to the goals set by the group as a whole or for the team of providers. They should include performance goals with targets and time deadlines. Each measure should also be very easily understood and be able to be changed regularly if they become easily achieved. Recognize successes with nonmonetary rewards and celebrations for the group or the team who showed achievement. Tell stories of team member successes to the whole group and begin to discover and tell stories of the values being brought to life and examples of how the new culture is becoming very real.

In a high-performing culture peers will begin to monitor each other as well as monitor the activities of the leaders. Leaders who can allow the top-down and the bottom-up flows of accountability and responsibility will be able to fully realize the way a high-performing culture works best. Also, leaders must be comfortable encouraging the empowerment of team leaders and individuals to have the authority and responsibility to make decisions based on metrics and values. Leaders of high-performing organizations also must have the courage to allow their people to have the freedom to fail. Always learning from failures and then moving forward. Attempts to avoid failure can be a very dangerous way to exist. Mistakes will happen with empowered teams; however, the lessons learned from these mistakes create an invaluable source of knowledge that lends to the high-performing culture we are seeking.

Leaders too must invest themselves in the development of the high-performing culture. They will need to invest meaningful time spent among team members, they will need to be visible, openly live the group's values, celebrate successes of the team, commit to living the values openly, and commit to never losing an "A" player. They will need to build communication systems with key messages, values stories of success, and make sure there is full commitment from all the senior leadership and the governance body [20].

A well-designed and implemented Values Blueprint positions the new culture for great success. Leaders get involved very early and demonstrate support for the new direction openly. Recruitment efforts for "A" players are intentional, new recruits are on-boarded with the core values from even before they accept employment, metrics for group and team performance are developed and made transparent, and lastly rewards and recognition programs are built to celebrate successes by the group. With this plan fully executed, a high-performing culture can be purposefully built in any organization, but it will never happen without hard work and focused dedication.

Building a Values-Based Culture: A Leadership Case Study

Hill Country Memorial Hospital (HCMH) is a nonprofit general acute care community hospital in the small rural town of Fredericksburg in the Texas Hill Country west of Austin. The hospital opened in 1971 and 93 % of the households in Gillespie County contributed financially to have it built. It serves approximately 3500 inpatients annually, performs over 4000 surgeries, handles more than 15,000 emergency department visits, performs more than 50,000 outpatient diagnostic and therapeutic procedures, cares for 350 Hospice patients and their loved ones at the end of life, and delivers over 500 new babies [21].

In 2010, like many rural hospitals, HCMH suffered from all three issues Don Berwick highlighted in his Triple Aim [15]. We had low patient satisfaction, low employee engagement, low employee satisfaction, deficient quality of care, poor financial performance, a disgruntled medical staff, and defensive legal posturing around patient complaints. With these facts staring us in the face. We decided to make a change. We knew to change our performance we must first change our culture.

In addition to Berwick, we had another strong influence on our goal to change our culture. We were both students of Peter Drucker, the iconic leadership and management author. We read many of his books and he influenced our goals and actions. Drucker said, "Organizations have to have values. But so do people. To be effective in an organization, one's own values must be compatible with the organization's values. They do not need to be the same. But they must be close enough so they can coexist. Otherwise the person will not produce results" [22]. We knew we wanted to change our results. It was time to change our culture.

In 2011, the 650-person team of Hill County Memorial Hospital set out on a journey to build a values-based culture. At the time, we had a list of stated values that hung proudly on our walls, but the ideas they represented were understood by only a few. We had taken no steps to ensure that our people's individual values were compatible with our stated organizational values. We decided to look for an evidenced-based solution to help us on our journey.

Having had a previous career where airline travel was the norm, I was very familiar with Southwest Airlines' simple culture based on three things: (1) get the customer where they want to go on time, (2) at the lowest possible fare, and (3) have a darn good time doing it. We studied Ann Rhoades' book *Built on Values* and came to understand our hospital team's values existed in the hearts and minds of our team members [15]. If we wanted to establish a values-based culture, it was first critical to understand the values that drove our team. Those values cannot be top driven from the C-Suite because those values drive behaviors, behaviors drive culture, and culture drives performance. We contacted Ann Rhoades and she agreed to help us on our journey. Ann assigned a small team headed by Gayle Watson to consult and guide us until we were well on our way.

We began our journey by forming a 31-person steering committee—a "values workout team." The team consisted of frontline team members from various hospital departments; members of each level of leadership; two physicians, and two patient family members. The family members' participation was critical to our process. One was the wife of a patient who died as a result of preventable harm *we* caused. The other was the father of a 13-year-old boy who died from a rare genetic condition. We treated the family horribly in the final days of the young man's life. In these two patient cases, we had already failed to meet two of Don Berwick's three aims to improve healthcare. We learned remarkable life lessons from these two families and it was important for us to have their input in building our culture and eventually changing the performance of the hospital. We are eternally grateful for their contribution.

We started the values workout session by asking each member of the team to write on paper his or her True North Values. The term comes from the book, *True North*, by Bill George, former Medtronic CEO, and refers to the internal moral compass each of us possesses that keeps us oriented on the right path [23]. What we wanted was for each member of the steering committee to develop a list of the values that drive them. We then asked team members to work in small groups of 5–6 people to determine a common list of values they all had in common. We repeated this for the group of 31. The result was a working list of six values with definitions of each one.

Next, our values workout team conducted listening tours throughout all hospital departments to get input from as many of our 650 HCM team members as possible. The input was extremely valuable and caused us to whittle from six to five common values shared by our entire team. We also made adjustments to the definition of one of our values. Compassion was defined by the committee as "Care for others with a joyful heart." Our Hospice team reminded us we cannot always have a joyful heart, but we can always be kind. We asked our entire HCM team to help us determine how we would know when we were living our values. This question prompted them to develop a list of behaviors to drive our culture.

On December 9, 2011, our values workout team leader presented "The *Remarkable* HCM Values" to the members of our Executive Team during our morning huddle (Fig. 7.2). She asked us to read them carefully. She then asked each of us to agree, on our honor, to abide by these values and behaviors developed by our team and use them to guide our key decisions. If we could not agree to do that, she asked us to resign from the HCM team. This moment, this question and our responses would determine if we were serious about changing our culture.

The C-Suite decided unanimously to support the values journey. This meant we each committed to hold ourselves accountable to the values and behaviors identified by the values workout team. It also meant we would be open to any team member holding us accountable when we veered off course. We also committed to holding others accountable. Accountability was the glue that held us all together. Establishing the values and behaviors was simply the first step along our journey. The hard work was about to begin.

Our next step was to align our values throughout our team. We used them as a screening tool to recruit new team members, leaders, physicians, and vendors. We used The *Remarkable* HCM Values as the basis of our leadership development program, the core of our quarterly coaching plans and to make difficult decisions affecting people and other critical resources. The *Remarkable* HCM Values were the foundation to our success and future sustainability.

THE *Remarkable* HCM VALUES

OTHERS FIRST
Commit to remarkable
care with each life
we touch

- Anticipates and exceeds expectations to deliver personalized service to patients, team members, family and friends.
- Listens and understands with empathy and a desire to understand thoughts, opinions and needs of others.
- Advocates teamwork.
- Embraces and honors individual diversity.
- Recognizes the contributions of others.
- Respects one another and the part they play in Hill Country Memorial's success.   **C**

COMPASSION
Care for others
with a kind heart

- Consistently treats others with courtesy, respect, kindness and patience.
- Shows genuine interest in what is important to others.
- Displays a helpful and friendly attitude.
- Supports and encourages through any situation.   **C**

INNOVATION
Integrate new
ideas with courage

- Embraces evidence based practices.
- Learns from experience and shares with others.
- Creates unique ways to provide remarkable care.
- Incorporates technology to improve patient and team member experience and outcomes.
- Thinks beyond the box.   **C**

ACCOUNTABILITY
Responsibility for
our actions

- Provides safe care.
- Leads by example at all times.
- Is open and honest about successes and failures.
- Takes initiative for own growth and development.
- Makes appropriate decisions in difficult situations.   **C**

STEWARDSHIP
Uphold our
responsibility for
lives & resources

- Demonstrates ownership of continuous improvement.
- Actively participates in our financial success by optimizing resources.
- Makes a positive contribution to the communities we serve.   **C**

C = COMMUNITY (our purpose and cornerstone)

☐ I have read and understand this document and, on my honor, agree to actively abide by The Remarkable HCM Values and behaviors detailed above.

Signature _____

Fig. 7.2 The remarkable HCM values, Hill Country Memorial Hospital, 2011

to change the culture of a 4000-person organization. We once again looked for a partner to help guide us.

We conducted a thorough, formal request for proposal process. We interviewed multiple companies. We found our partner—People Ink, Inc. led by Ann Rhoades and Gayle Watson. People Ink's mission is to help organizations create unique cultures based on values and performance. Ann is the author of the book, *Built on Values* [26]. She helped us understand the relationship between leaders, values, culture, and performance: Leaders drive values. Values drive behaviors. Behaviors drive culture. And culture drives performance. If we want to change our culture we need to first identify the core values of the people in our organization and we need leaders who will drive those values that will, in turn, drive the specific behaviors our team expects.

Our values steering committee worked with Gayle Watson and Shannon Mick of People Ink, Inc. to develop a survey and focus groups. We wanted to better understand our current culture. We had a 60 % response rate from the survey. We also had 300 team members attend very active focus group sessions. The team's message came through loud and clear. We asked, "Does our organization have a list of stated values?" Almost everyone said "yes." We then asked respondents to name them. Less than 1 % of those answering the survey could name our values. We have them, but we aren't living them in a meaningful way for our team. We also learned that we have a general lack of trust of leaders and each other. Over and over, we heard comments of "fear of retaliation and retribution." We wanted to make a change. We needed to make a change if we want to improve our performance.

Our next step was to form a diverse Values Team whose charter was to develop a list of common core values we all share. A list that each team member could see and say, "That's me." We identified 50 people representing all our organizational departments. We selected as diverse a team as we could put together. We wanted people who think differently and have the courage to speak out—to represent themselves and others. Among the team we had three community members who we trust.

We gathered off campus for a 2-day session and our UNTHSC President opened the session with his vision for us to develop a values-based culture whose foundation is trust.

Next we explained the concept of *True North*, as written by Bill George in his book of the same name [23]. True North refers to the idea that inside each one of us is an internal moral compass. The North arrow of the compass points to the values and principles we hold so dear we will not compromise them to stay in a job or a relationship. These are the values that define us.

Once each of us wrote down our values, we then shared them with our table-mates. The goal was to create a list at each table that reflected just the values we share. Each of us might have other values we hold dear but are not common to the team. While these are important because they help define us as individuals, our task was to develop a list of those we all share—our organizational True North. Each table group had a list it displayed and we then looked around the room to identify the themes that emerged. We had a lively debate and in the end identified our draft of common core values—Serve Others First, Integrity, Respect, Collaboration, and Be Visionary. We added definitions for each value and most importantly five behaviors for each so we will know when we are living our values.

We held 67 listening tours in departments throughout the organization and made adjustments to the definitions and behaviors. Everyone had the ability to propose changes. We incorporated the recommendations into the final document and released Our Values to the team in September 2014 (Fig. 7.3).

Our next step was to focus on our leadership. We want to develop a leadership team who extends trust to our team and in return earns their trust. Again we sought help from an expert. Several of us had read and were greatly impressed by Stephen M.R. Covey's book, *Speed of Trust* [27]. A few of us traveled to meet Stephen and hear him speak.

In November 2014, Mike who was now the UNTHSC President recorded a video emphasizing his point that trust is the foundation of our values [28]. He also summarized the major lessons we learned from Stephen. In the video, he defines Covey's four elements of building and maintaining trust—integrity, intent, capabilities, and results. He ends by giving us his commitment to build a new culture whose foundation is trust.

The Office of People Development organized a monthly leadership program for the top 125 leaders in the organization. We called the program Leadership 125 (L125) and our goal was to work together to study the Thirteen Behaviors of a High Trust Leader that Stephen M.R. Covey details in his book. We named our theme for 2015 as "Leading at the Speed of Trust."

We published a leader's *Field Guide* designed for leaders to carry and use. It summarizes what we learned together. My hope is we continue to work together to extend our trust and build our values-based culture. We are on a journey. Please join us. We hope you will find that by focusing first on establishing a values-based culture, you will be able to create a high-performing team.

Conclusion

Core values-based culture change and transformation to a high-performing organization can happen with intention and purpose. It requires leaders who are willing to commit to the core values and live them openly by displaying the defined behaviors for each value. Focused, humble, and committed leaders can drive values throughout an entire group of providers if they do it with purpose and with the best intentions for the group as a whole. Once the frontline team buys into the same idea of a values-based culture and they go through the process of building the Values Blueprint the foundation has been laid. With values developed and behaviors defined the culture begins to be created. Leaders and team members commit openly to living the values each and every day. Stories of the values being lived out and celebrated begin to be commonplace inside the culture. Decisions are made more easily, providers are empowered to make decisions for the group, and the group becomes more nimble to unexpected challenges. It becomes fun to go to work each and every day and look for the best ways to take care of customers (patients and their families). Peers support peers and leaders

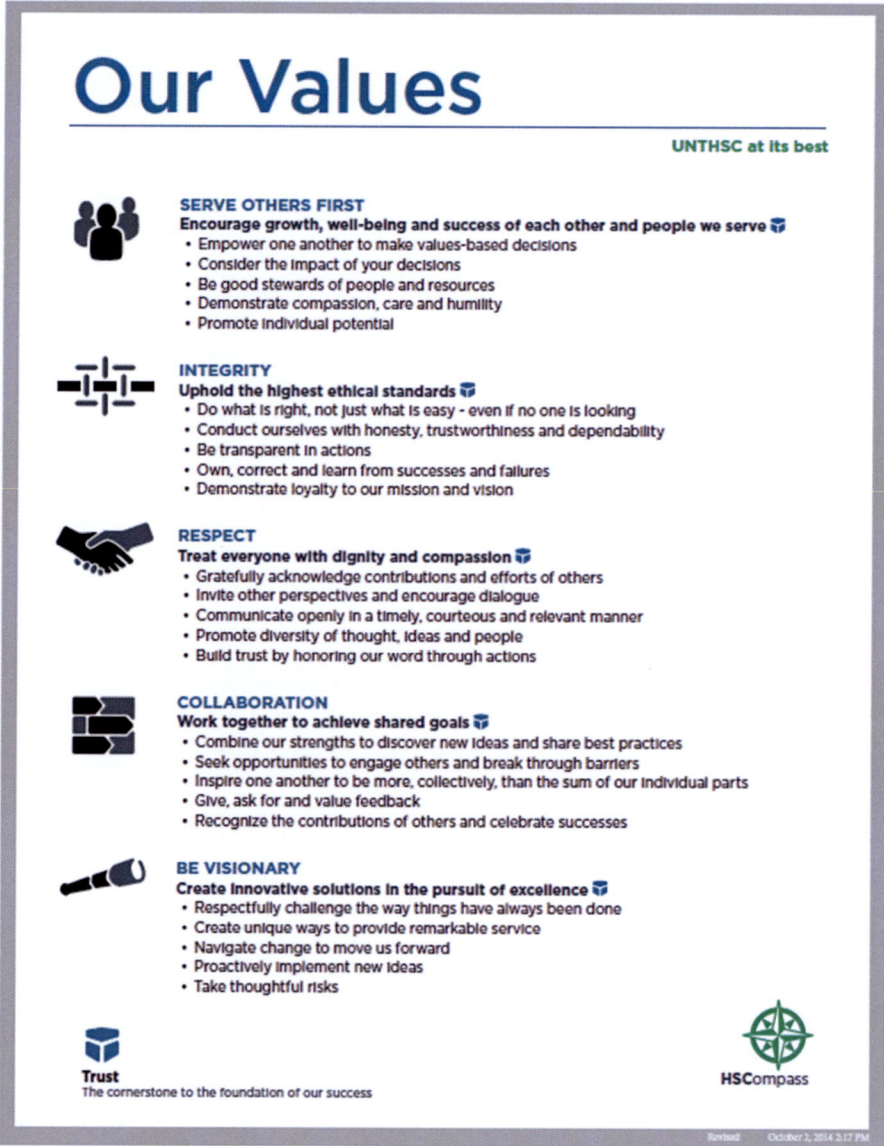

Fig. 7.3 Our values—the University of North Texas Health Center Culture of Care

support the entire team. Communication occurs in two directions, from top to bottom and bottom to top. Trust quickly builds and is easily sustained with the openly visible living of values inside and outside the organization. Earlier in this chapter we said that integrity is the concept of being consistent in your behaviors, consistent in your core values and the methods used to reach your goals. The values-based, high-performing culture we described throughout this chapter is a culture of very high integrity and trust. People want to work for this type of group, patients want to be cared for by this type of group, and no one wants to go elsewhere once they have experienced it. It is a purposeful journey and one worth the hard work and struggle to achieve it. Those who would oppose it are simply those who will always fight to guard the status quo, complacency, or mediocrity they have become so comfortable in. We challenge you to join us and take on the fight to create such a culture in your provider group. It is the right thing to do for your people, organization, and your customers!

References

1. Disney R. Available from BrainyQuote.com http://www.brainyquote.com/quotes/quotes/r/royedisne170949.html (n.d.). Accessed 31 December 2015.
2. Simpson A. Quoted by Gergen D. in Eyewitness to power: the essence of leadership Nixon to Clinton. New York: Simon & Schuster; 2001.
3. Souba WW. Academic medicine's core values: what do they mean? J Surg Res. 2003;115:171–3.
4. Pellegrino ED. Physician integrity, why it is inviolable. Connecting American values with health reform. The Hastings Center. p. 18–20.
5. Rasayon J. Why you shouldn't confuse physician employment with alignment. The Advisory Board Company; 2015.
6. Rhoades A, Shepherdson N. Built on values. San Francisco: Jossey-Bass; 2011. p. 15.
7. Integrity [Definition 1–3] in Merriam-Webster Online. Available from http://www.merriam-webster.com/dictionary/integrity. (n.d.). Accessed 27 December 2015.
8. Integrity [Definition 1] in Merriam-Webster Online. Available from http://www.merriam-webster.com/dictionary/integrity. (n.d.). Accessed 27 December 2015.
9. Integrity [Definition 2] in Merriam-Webster Online. Available from http://www.merriam-webster.com/dictionary/integrity. (n.d.). Accessed 27 December 2015.
10. Integrity [Definition 3] in Merriam-Webster Online. Available from http://www.merriam-webster.com/dictionary/integrity. (n.d.). Accessed 27 December 2015.
11. Leader [Definition 2a] in Merriam-Webster Online. Available from www.merriam-webster.com/dictionary/leader. (n.d.). Accessed 27 December 2015.
12. Guide [Simple Definition] in Merriam-Webster Online. Available from http://www.merriam-webster.com/dictionary/guide. (n.d.). Accessed 27 December 2015.
13. Conductor [Medical Definition 2] in Merriam-Webster Online. Available from http://www.merriam-webster.com/dictionary/conductor. (n.d.). Accessed 27 December 2015.
14. Robert Galvin interview: 'a deficiency of will and ambition': a conversation with Donald Berwick. Health Affairs; January 2005.
15. Berwick DM, Nolan TW, Whittington J. The triple aim: care, health, and cost. Health Affairs; May/June 2008.
16. Behavior [Definition 1c] in Merriam-Webster Online. Available from www.merriam-webster.com/dictionary/leader. (n.d.). Accessed 28 December 2015.
17. Rhoades A, Shepherdson N. Built on values. San Francisco: Jossey-Bass; 2011. p. 13.
18. Drucker P. Reply-mc.com. Available from http://www.reply-mc.com/people/peter-drucker/. Accessed 31 December 2015.
19. Rhoades A, Shepherdson N. Built on values. San Francisco: Jossey-Bass; 2011. p. 33–50.
20. Rhoades A, Shepherdson N. Built on values. San Francisco: Jossey-Bass; 2011. p. 39, 133.
21. Hill Country Memorial Hospital Malcolm Baldrige national quality award application; 2013.
22. Drucker P. What are my values? The essential Drucker. New York: HarperCollins; 2011. p. 223.

23. George B, Sims P. True North: discover your authentic leadership. San Francisco: Jossey-Bass; 2007. p. xxiii, xxiv, xxxv.
24. Truven Healthcare Analytics, 100 top hospital rankings, as reported at http://100tophospitals.com/studies-winners/100-top-hospitals/year/2015.
25. Women's Choice Awards as reported at: http://www.womenschoiceaward.com/awarded/best-hosp/featured/hill-country-memorial-hospital/.
26. Rhoades A, Shepherdson N. Built on values. San Francisco: Jossey-Bass; 2011. p. v–vii.
27. Covey SMR, Merrill R. The speed of trust: the one thing that changes everything. New York: Free Press; 2006.
28. Williams M. Trust is a Must video, published 19 November 2014. www.YouTube.com. Available from: https://www.youtube.com/watch?v=X2UcGtADNrE.

Chapter 8
Perspectives from Single Payer Systems

Eyal Zimlichman and Yishay Falick

Introduction

While generally health care in the United States has shown improvement in performance metrics with isolated demonstrations of improving value for patients, the main crises remain inflated costs that threaten to become unsustainable. With Americans spending almost 18 % of their Gross Domestic Product (GDP) on health care, one cannot overlook the striking dissimilarity to other developed countries that spend sometimes half as much and yet demonstrate similar and sometimes improved performance and outcomes. This remarkable fact requires us to dig in and better understand how this is attained, and more importantly, what can be learned for the U.S. so that similar achievements are made: both on the National and policymakers' level, as well as on the payer and provider level.

We tend to regard free markets as the basis for a healthy competition-driven environment where the consumer is the main beneficiary as costs go down while value for consumer increases. The health care market in the U.S. has traditionally followed that concept, yet cost reductions have not been achieved and value has not followed the patients. Due to characteristics unique to health care, we now understand that free markets need to be regulated in a fashion that would allow for continuous cost control as well as drive patient centered value.

Single payer health care markets are blossoming outside the U.S. and are generally associated with better outcomes at lower costs. Medical care expenditures and

E. Zimlichman, M.D., M.Sc. (✉)
Central Management, Sheba Medical Center,
Tel Hashomer, Ramat Gan 5265601, Israel
e-mail: Eyal.zimlichman@sheba.health.gov.il

Y. Falick, M.D., M.B.A.
Department of Medical Affairs, Ministry of Health,
Jerusalem 9101002, Israel

© Springer International Publishing Switzerland 2017
H.C. Sax (ed.), *Measurement and Analysis in Transforming Healthcare Delivery*, DOI 10.1007/978-3-319-46222-6_8

life expectancy, for example, on average among countries in the Organization for Economic Cooperation and Development (OECD) have been favorable compared to the U.S. [1]. The "capitalist" oriented notion that single payer systems lack the inherent competition needed to improve consumer-oriented value thus needs to be questioned.

In this chapter, the origin and structure of single payer systems relating to the stakeholders, the payment systems, and quality metrics and programs will be described. We will then describe in details a case study of the Israeli Health care system, a single payer system which has achieved impressive cost containment through regulations yet managed to drive improvement through competition. Finally, we will try to draw lessons that might be applicable to policymakers, providers, and payers in the U.S.

Structure of Single Payer Systems

Single payer health care system is the term used to describe the funding mechanism of health care services by a single public body which collects all medical fees, then pays for all services. The aim of this system is to provide universal (or near universal) health care coverage. Different countries utilize various types of delivery, either owning health care resources and services or contracting them from private organizations. Either way the fees for all health care services are paid by this public source and not by private insurers.

The funding in this health insurance model comes from the covered population (citizens and legal residents). Yet, in some cases people get coverage despite exemption from payment. The government can either manage the program directly or use publicly owned and regulated bodies. Among the benefits of employing single payer systems are its relative administrative simplicity, vast population coverage, and cost control by various methods such as obtaining lower prices from suppliers as a result of the enormous market power, setting fixed service prices, and controlling the supply of health services.

Nowadays many country's health care systems are based on mixed elements from three historically distinguished single payer models: Beveridge, Bismarck, and National health insurance models. The historical backgrounds, as well as current sociopolitical and economic status of each country influence the magnitude of implementation of each element in this complex system. We will describe these models briefly in order to get a better understanding of their components.

The Beveridge Model—The Beveridge Report (1943) was the basis for the "welfare state" in post WWII Britain. On these foundations the National Health Service (NHS) act (1946) has been legislated. The core principle for this system regards health as a universal human right, mandating health coverage as a legal right. In a Pure Beveridgean system, as implemented in Cuba, the country provides medical care for free, based on need rather than on one's ability to pay. Financed by taxation the rich contributes more than the poor. The government owns most hospitals and clinics and is one of the main employers of doctors. All health providers collect their fees from the government and both citizens and residents are eligible for treatment at any institution anywhere in the country.

The Bismarck Model—As part of the unification of Germany Bismarck formed the welfare state, mandating "Social Health Insurance" in 1883. This insurance-based model is still in use in Germany and has been adopted by Japan and other countries utilizing preexisting "sickness funds." The core principle for this system associates the right for health with labor status and regard health as a privilege. This model goal is to improve productivity, preempt labor unrest by maintaining workers health, and is not aiming for universal coverage for all citizens and residents. Funds are collected by a compulsory employers' and employees' payroll deduction. The population insured is entitled for health services offered mostly by private sector providers and by the state.

The National Health Insurance Model—A universal health care insurance program is run by the government. Canada and Taiwan are some examples. As in the Beveridge system this program is financed by universal taxation and covers every citizen and resident. However, this insurance program pays for both public and private sector providers as in the Bismarck model.

The Out-of-Pocket Model—In the pure form of this model, medical fees are paid directly to the provider or to the insurer by the consumer. Both lack of control over private health care supplier's rates and consumer low market power tend to lead to higher prices, lower population coverage, and reduce use of services and access to them. As insurance is supplied by private agents they often use "cherry picking" insuring healthier populations and avoiding sicker ones. The basic rule in such system is that the richer get better medical care and the poorer gets worse treatment if they get any at all.

In single payer health care markets, policy and regulations are critical to allow for the improvement of quality and control of costs. The single payer can form joint ventures with stakeholders such as professional organizations/unions, accreditation bodies, and patient groups to achieve mutual goals. For this aim the single payer utilizes his vast influence and control over other stakeholders such as insurance companies, providers, and pharmaceutical companies. The single payer control over rates of nearly all health care goods and services may help to contain costs even in a fee for service settings. Japan as a case study proves that despite lower rate of health spending meticulous government regulation can maintain access to care, avoid rationing, make use of the latest technology, and show impressive health measures results [2].

Nonsingle payer systems tend to increase cost as they lack central control over provider rates and "fee for service" generate suppliers-induced demand as a result of economic incentive to "sell" more services such as costly procedures. There is accumulative data supporting favorable results to pay for performance programs implemented by single payer over those implemented by nonsingle payer. In a large-scale study the long-term effect of hospital pay for performance initiative on mortality showed that in a region of England adoption of a specific quality program, based on the largest implemented program in the U.S., has led to a clinically significant reduction in 30-day in-hospital mortality during the first 18 months [3]. In the following 24 months, mortality continued to decline but to a lesser extent. Moreover, the effect in England has been more positive than in the United States. Among other reasons the authors attributed this difference to the fact that a single payer has better control over issues such as the universal participation of hospitals and the collaborative nature of the initiative. Similarly, smaller studies showed favorable results for single payer "pay for outcome" programs such as increasing the effectiveness and supply of smoking cessation services [4].

Community quality improvement programs implemented by single payer tend to be successful because of sufficient allocation of resources. Such was the case in the breast screening program implemented by the NHS in the UK [5].

The advantage of having a single payer system in regard to quality metrics is its ability to form a comprehensive performance framework which aligns with the broader strategic goals and priorities of the health care system. Such framework enables monitoring and reporting on health care system performance which will lay the foundations for health reform over time.

A comparison between leading OECD countries which utilizes single payer system versus the USA with its mixed health care system based mostly on private sector providers and insurers found disadvantage to the latter exhibiting shorter life expectancy and higher infant mortality despite spending on average twice as much on health as demonstrated by its health expenditure in percentage from GDP. Furthermore, when comparing such measures related to chronic disease management and measures of hospitalization for conditions such as asthma, chronic obstructive pulmonary disease (COPD), congestive heart failure, and diabetes, the U.S. again shows lower rates compared to OECD single payer system countries such as the U.K., Japan, Canada, and Israel [1, 6].

The Case of the Israeli Health Care System

The health care system in Israel is one of contrasts: social foundations yet highly competitive market, low cost spending (half the average of OECD countries) yet continuously improving population health outcomes and high quality community health care services with hospital care catching up. The reforms that have helped shape this unique system stem back to the foundations of the State of Israel, although the last 20 years have seen a new set of reforms centered around: equity, patient rights and patient centric care, national quality measurement at the community level and now also at the hospital level, and quality and patient safety national initiatives aiming to further improve performance (Table 8.1).

The Israeli Health Care System

The broader health care system stems from social foundations set in place when the State of Israel was established in 1948. As a result, the current structure is primarily tax funded, based largely on State activities. Universal coverage is provided to all citizens and permanent residents through a national health insurance system that

Table 8.1 Comparing Israel and the United States on key attributes

Attribute	Israel	United States
Source of finance	Government, out of pocket	Employers, government, out of pocket
Percent insured	100	85
Percent managed care	100	25–35
Physician reimbursement	Primary care—salary and capitation	Fee for service
	Hospital—salary	Growing pay for performance
Per capita spending on health care (US$) [1]	2428	8713
Infant mortality rate (per 1000 live births) [1]	2.5	5.0
Average life span at birth (years) [1]	Men—80.3	Men—76.4
	Women—83.9	Women—81.2

allows the insured to choose a health plan. Income-based health tax is collected through the National Insurance Agency and distributed to the health plans per capita of insured individuals and adjusted for age, gender, and geographical parameters. The four nonprofit, competing health plans (Clalit, Maccabi, Meuhedet, and Leumit) must provide their members with access to a benefits package that is specified in the national law, also providing community health care services to all citizens [7]. Citizens/residents can transfer from one Health Fund to another up to two times a year and cannot be refused coverage. Although only a small number actually transfer between Health Plans (1.5 % as of 2009) this mechanism is the driving force that promotes competition between the Health Plans who are competing for every individual. Although there are a few private hospitals, most acute care beds and long-term inpatient facilities are operated by the government, and the government sets the level of per capita financing that all four health plans receive. Clalit (the largest health plan that insures roughly 50 % of the population) is the only health plan to run its own hospitals, operating about one-third of the general hospitals in the country. Patients can approach any general hospital for emergency and acute conditions, while for elective admissions; the Health Plan would refer to a specific hospital, generally with whom they would have a favorable contract with.

Recent years have seen policy reforms around quality and patient safety. The government, and specifically the Ministry of Health (MOH), is charged with the responsibility to reform Israel's health care system and address the above-mentioned challenges. Yet, much of the initiatives impacting quality and safety have originated from the health plans that have individually set the agenda ahead of national policy. Such is the case for setting a national community quality indicators program (and later for hospitals), large-scale patient experience surveys, and policy for the accreditation of general hospitals (Clalit were the first to contract with the Joint Commission International for accreditation services, later this became mandatory by the MOH).

National quality indicators programs started relatively late in Israel. In 2004 the Israel National Institute for Health Policy and Health Services Research launched the National Program for Quality Indicators in Community Healthcare in Israel (QICH). With the intention of being able to compare across countries, indicators were based on existing international measures, mostly from the Healthcare Effectiveness Data and Information Set (HEDIS) of the National Committee for Quality Assurance (NCQA) in the United States. With all four health plans cooperating and supporting the program, it was considered a success from its early days and has demonstrated continuous improvement since. The program was designed to allow comparison of performance indicators across countries. As Rosen et al. have found, in a comparative analysis of adherence to standards of care between Israel and the United States, Israel achieves comparable quality on several primary care indicators but with more rapid quality improvement [8].

Measuring quality of care in hospitals started much later with the MOH stepping in and filling the gap only in 2012. The National Program for Quality Indicators in Hospitals currently includes about 50 process measures which are reported by general, psychiatric, and geriatric hospitals to the MOH. Following a robust validation process performed by the MOH, quality measures are publically reported, usually drawing much public attention.

Within the Israeli health care system another key player is the Israeli Medical Association (IMA) which represents the physicians in Israel and acts both as a workers union and in setting and overseeing professional standards for physician's specialization programs. This duality poses a potential for a conflict between representing the physician's interests and ensuring high quality and safety. This will be discussed in more detail later in this chapter.

Doctor and nurses are employed by the hospital. Physician salary is low compared to other OECD countries, demanding doctors to work after hours in either an outpatient clinic for one of the health plans or performing procedures at one of the private for-profit hospitals.

Mechanisms of Cost Containment

To reach a state in which national health care expenditures as part of the GDP are half the OECD average demands considerable cost containment strategies set by the government, under the control of the Israeli Ministry of Finance. A national health care "basket" is defined by law and set at a fixed monetary amount adjusted annually by the health care cost index. About 2 % of the health care national budget is set each year for emerging technologies (mostly pharmaceuticals) where a committee convened annually decides which new technologies would be included in the health "basket." Yet, the health care budget is eroding from year to year due to the natural growth of the population and the fact that there is no adjustment to population health status and comorbidities.

Most of the health care budget is distributed to the Health Plans directly on an annual basis based on a per-capita allocation system (adjusted for age, gender, and socioeconomic status). This represents 88 % of the income for the Health Plans (as of 2014). The Health Plans rely heavily on this subsidy and focus much of their efforts on recruiting new members. The hospitals are payed by the Health Plans mostly on a fee for service approach—either through a differential payment system (similar in many respects to the Diagnosis Related Groups (DRG) system) for elective procedures, or on a per-diem (per day) method for nonelective hospitalizations. Charge for differential payments and charge per in-hospital day is set by the government (a joint ministry of finance and ministry of health committee) and is updated in accordance with the public wage index and the consumer price index. Yet, these set charges are also eroded to a point where prices do not reflect actual cost. This is a major contributing factor leading to the reality in which most hospitals in Israel, on one hand, are losing money on a yearly basis, but on the other hand find themselves constantly innovating in an effort to become more efficient as well as look for new revenue streams. Furthermore, payment mechanisms exist that encourage control of referrals for elective procedures to the hospitals. This is done through a capping mechanism set by the government that sets lower prices (not profitable) as volume increases so as to provide disincentives for the hospitals to accept higher patient volumes. This is of course different than what is often seen in the U.S. health care market where hospitals set discounted, yet still profitable, prices for higher volumes—creating an incentive to increase referral rates and inflate health care utilization and spending. Still, the Health Plans in Israel struggle financially and as for FY2012–2014, two of the four have showed a deficit of up to 2 % of total revenues.

Incentives and Disincentives for Performance Improvement

Before a summary of incentives for performance improvement is provided, it is essential to understand the disincentive forces that exist in the Israeli health care system, as an example of a single payer system. First of all, since the state has the responsibility to care for the residents and since the system as a whole is working with very little potential for excess capacity, hospitals and health plans must continue to operate, almost regardless of financial status. Indeed, the state will cover losses through various mechanisms at the end of the fiscal year. This is very common for the government-owned hospitals but also happens with the health plans and even other public hospitals (such as the case with Hadassah Medical Center in Jerusalem that has survived through a major financial crises through intense government subsidy). This, of course, provides a disincentive for hospitals (and to some extent the health plans) to drive for financial stability and profitability. Lack of clear incentives to improve financial outcomes also contributes to disincentives for quality improvement.

From a policy point of view, very little reimbursement is tied to quality. Apart from within the Clalit health fund, which operates both hospitals and community services, other hospitals have virtually no incentive to prevent readmissions, for example. Indeed, Clalit hospitals have implemented a successful continuity of care program that has resulted in substantial reduction in readmission rates, yet this did not spread to other health plans or to government-owned hospitals. Still, potentially avoidable readmission rates are generally better than in the U.S. [9].

When referring to improving performance of individual physicians, it is challenging to identify incentive methods within the public health care system in Israel. For one, salaries are set and financial bonuses tied to performance are not allowed. So performance cannot be tied to financial gains. This is of course similar to other health care sectors working within the public systems in Israel such as nursing. Furthermore, to complicate matters, the Israeli Medical Association, acting as both a union for physicians but also as a policy body setting the standards for physicians, is limiting the use of individual performance assessment and feedback perceived by them as a threat to physician's interests. Of course, preventing feedback based on performance assessment, benchmarking, and identifying best practices, as well as decreasing variability between providers, are all critical elements for quality improvement. National medical associations often play a role in improving quality on a national scale through either setting guidelines, quality measures and benchmark, and/or laying down a system for continuous medical education [10–12]. While in Israel the IMA does play a role mostly through setting professional guidelines and professional regulation of residency programs, in its perceived role as a union, some actions are regarded as a barrier to further performance improvement.

With all the challenges and difficulties to create meaningful incentive programs, how is improvement in performance gained and sustained in the Israeli health care systems? The (surprising) answer in one word would be "competition."

Health Plans

Competition between the health plans is fundamental since payment by the government is being done per person insured and residents can switch between the plans. This brings about a "race" to reach and register every potential enrollee. Indeed the health plans are spending increasing amounts on improving the patient experience as well as on marketing and advertisement campaigns. All four plans have gone through an organizational cultural change with focus on the patient experience and patient-centered care during the early 2000 years, as a response to the National Health Insurance Law in 1995 and the Patient's Rights Law in 1996. National patient experience surveys have generally registered high and improving scores across the plans [13]. The National Program for Quality Indicators in Community Healthcare in Israel has been publically reporting 50 quality measures comparatively for the four health plans since 2010. This has led to continuous improvement on multiple measures relating to cancer screening, cardiovascular care, diabetes, and other chronic disease management.

When comparing quality indicators in the community longitudinally a significant improvement can be seen in many of the indicators. Jaffe et al. have done a comparison across 3 years (2006–2009) and demonstrated an overall improvement, especially in proper documentation and to a lesser extent in other indicators such as primary prevention measures and documentation of cardiovascular risk [14]. It is believed that the relationship between the launch of the National Program for Quality Indicators in the Community and the improvement in the performance is causative. It is clear that the health plans have taken seriously the quality measurement and have invested in improvement programs and restructuring as well as continuously tracking their performance on a district level as well as a practice level.

As Rosen et al. have found, in a comparative analysis of adherence to standards of care between Israel and the United States, Israel achieves comparable quality on several primary care indicators and more rapid quality improvement [15]. While for adherence to screening standards Israel was lagging behind the U.S., in adherence to standards for care of diabetes patients the compliance in Israel was higher. In terms of intermediate outcomes achieved, in Israel the rate of uncontrolled diabetes was lower (13.3 % vs. 31.0 % in the U.S. patients with A1c Hb above 9 %) and the rate of controlled hypertension was higher (66.8 % vs. 31.7 %, respectively, with systolic blood pressure under 130 mmHg) [8]. Similar to the experience from the U.S., it seems that the true effect of public reporting of measures is through the actions of the providers themselves, while changes in consumer preference are limited [15].

Hospitals

Performance improvement in hospitals as well as continuous quality measurement has been more sporadic until the MOH quality reforms were initiated in 2011/2012. Specifically these refer to the National Program for Hospital Quality Measures as well as the policy on accreditation of acute care and later psychiatric hospitals by the Joint Commission International (JCI). In 2009, cross sectional surveys performed by the MOH have found gaps in various performance measures in acute care hospitals. These include performance on time-sensitive issues such as treatment of STEMI (ST elevation myocardial infarction), surgery for hip fractures, and treatment of acute stroke, as well as for timely administration of prophylactic antibiotics prior to surgery. These gaps, together with the OECD report in 2012 criticizing hospital care in Israel for its nontransparency, led the MOH to set much-needed policy reforms. The next few years have seen much-needed improvement as hospitals built quality and patient safety foundations and embarked on continuous quality improvement programs. Public reporting of quality measures had a key role in the success of these processes. Again, similar to the health plans, competition between hospitals was a major factor in driving improvement. But this was not so much with aim of increasing patient volumes but rather due to the competition between hospitals for perceived professionalism, prestige, and inherent strive for excellence.

How are these improvements achieved in an environment where financial incentives are not possible and physician level metrics are not used as a driver for improvement? A key component would be leadership, both clinical as well as from management. The inherent professional competition is likely on two levels—between hospitals as a whole but also between similar services in different hospitals. So while CEOs of hospital A and hospital B are competing on which is a better hospital, chief of cardiology, for example, in hospital A and chief of cardiology in hospital B are competing on which is the better service. The impact of leadership on performance improvement is critical in Israel, specifically regarding clinical leadership. One of the reasons for this would be the central role of the clinical chief or the department director. The chiefs play a central role in the clinical policy, control, staff appointments, teaching, and research activities within the service or department. They are more autonomous when compared to their counterparts in the U.S. and thus are also typically more competitive.

Another contributing factor to performance improvement is the fact that all physicians are employed by the hospital as physician groups are nonexistent in Israel. This increases considerably the sense of belonging and identity with the hospital and also the sense of motivation and competitiveness. Under the right leadership at both the hospital level, as well as the service/department level, striving for performance improvement, the sense of identity would be a contributing factor. The alignment of interests and incentives between hospital and staff, and between the different sectors in the hospitals, all employed by the same employer, allows for easier control, clinical integration, and launching of improvement programs.

Although it was only recently launched, the National Program for Hospital Quality Measures has already showed quick improvement across all measures. This is attributable to the public reporting as annually the MOH releases results for all hospitals in what become a well-communicated public event. Some of the gaps measured in 2009 were rapidly closing. Prophylactic antibiotics in a 1 h window prior to colon surgery went up from 44 % nationwide in 2009 to 82 % and 86 % in 2013 and 2014, respectively. Surgery performed within 48 h for hip fracture went up from 63 % nationwide in 2009 to 77 % and 80 % in 2013 and 2014, respectively. Currently, the MOH National Program for Hospital Quality Measures includes 20 measures for acute care hospitals, 15 measures for geriatric hospitals, and 14 measures for psychiatric hospitals. Still, as of the writing of this chapter, all measures are process measures with no outcome measures included so far (plans exist to measure and report health care acquired infections in 2016). It is our expectations that once outcomes are measured and reported through the program, rapid improvements would also be seen. When referring to these improvements in both hospital care and community health care, Dr. Mark Chassin, president and chief executive officer of The Joint Commission, stated that "These accomplishments are all the more impressive given Israel's modest overall per capita spending on health care, and because they apply, with very few exceptions, to the entire population of the country" [16]. Indeed, Israel makes it seem possible to curb cost of health care in a single-payer regulated environment *and* observe concurrent meaningful increase in quality.

Lessons Learned from Single Payer Systems

It seems that single payer systems are succeeding in what is considered by many to be the Holy Grail: improving health care for populations and improving hospital-based performance while restraining health care costs. Taking a close look at the Israeli health care system as an example can teach us a few lessons both at the national policy level as well as at the provider level.

Table 8.2 Key lessons learned from single-payer systems to allow improving quality and controlling cost of health care

Structural/policy factors	Further proliferation of integrated health care systems with vertical integration of providers (also through accountable care organizations)
	Wide adoption of electronic medical records with health information exchange between all levels of care
	Tight cost control and capping of payments for services through more managed care
	Mergers of hospital systems with centralized decision making and resource budgeting
Provider initiated factors	Strengthen clinical leadership and accountability for performance
	Leverage inherent professional competition for reputation and status, especially among academic medical centers
	Adopt a "hospital employed physicians" model rather than physician organization to align goals and incentives
	Develop and use real-time quality and operational metrics through system-wide control systems (business intelligence dashboards)

Obviously there are important structural differences between Israel and the U.S. that are unlikely to change in the near future. These include the single payer nature of course but also the relatively small share of health maintenance organizations; the scattering of care among many more health plans; and the lack of a common, unifying national framework. However, a few conclusions from this review could potentially be relevant and serve as recommendations for the U.S. health care system (Table 8.2).

On the macro/structural level—single payer markets certainly can sustain successful competition. Both between health plans but also between hospitals, whether they are government owned or owned by the health plan. Combined with public reporting of performance metrics competition will drive improvement in service and quality. Regulations that are part of a national framework can pose strict cost control, through tight budgets and capping of payments to providers.

Yet structural differences are presumably just part of the success of single payer systems. Similarities can be seen to the successful transformation of a U.S.-based single payer system, the Veterans Affairs (VA), in the mid-1990s. The VA too had comparable elements such as the VA's centralized decision-making capabilities, salaried physician workforce, educational programs, and fixed capped budgets. It took reorganization on multiple fronts to drive the transformation. Although these included implementation of a systematic approach to the measurement of, management of, and accountability for quality, it was also goal setting and resource budgeting on a central level that likely drove improvement [17]. We believe this approach would be similar in the case of the Israeli health care system and could be a factor in promoting quality while controlling costs.

On the community level, Israel's achievements can partially be explained through the integration of care and strong alignment of incentives between insurance and providers. In the U.S. this is relatively similar to integrated health care systems in which vertical integration (linking different levels of care, e.g., primary, secondary, and tertiary care) takes place. Similar to the health plans in Israel, the wide adoption of electronic medical records across the system (with effective use of decision support tools) would allow seamless integration between all care levels [18]. In integrated managed care the insurance is part of the health plan and this is where most incentives converge and allow for cost containment achieved mainly through better care in the community, improved population health, and improved care for chronically ill patients. The proliferation of accountable care organizations (ACO) and bundled payments are all similar concepts aimed toward more integrated managed care [19].

What can we learn from single payer systems to drive improved performance within hospitals? As we have seen in the Israeli case example, competition between hospitals is still a major driving force for improvement even in a non-for-profit environment, and even when patient volumes are regulated through payment capping mechanisms. This is attributable to the inherent professional competition for reputation and status among hospitals, particularly academic medical centers. Leveraging competition and reputation to drive performance improvement requires strong leadership and accountability from the CEO as well as the clinical directors. The importance of leadership and the driving force of competition among institutions have also played a factor in the VA transformation [20]. Here too, information technology was an important enabler, specifically real-time quality as well as operational metrics and business intelligence dashboards customized for use by the clinical directors as well as hospital management. As is the case with Israel and the VA, employing physicians by the hospitals helps in continuous performance improvement through alignment of goals and incentives.

Summary

In this chapter, we have attempted to review single payer systems, mostly from an international perspective, and highlight some of the achievements, specifically in regards to advancing quality while controlling costs in a level that is sometimes superior to that achieved in the U.S. Although structurally different, lessons can still be picked up from single payer systems on local and international.

One of the key issues demonstrated through the example of the Israeli health care system is the importance of competition between health funds as well as between hospitals, a competition which is just as fierce as it is in a for-profit market or a multipayer system. This competition enables services to be more patient centered and drives performance improvement. Furthermore, we believe that a policy of public reporting, continuous measurement, and accountability in an integrated managed care environment are keys to control costs while allowing for improving performance. Building clinical leadership on all levels and use of information technology both as integrated one-stop-shop medical record and also as management control tools are both necessary to allow any medical system to be effective, efficient, and sustainable.

References

1. Health at a Glance. OECD indicators. Paris: OECD Publishing; 2015. http://dx.doi.org/10.1787/health_glance-2015-en.
2. Ikegami N, Anderson GF. In Japan, all-payer rate setting under tight government control has proved to be an effective approach to containing costs. Health Aff (Millwood). 2012;31(5):1049–56.
3. Kristensen SR, Meacock R, Turner AJ, Boaden R, McDonald R, Roland M, Sutton M. Long-term effect of hospital pay for performance on mortality in England. N Engl J Med. 2014;371(6):540–8.
4. McLeod H, Blissett D, Wyatt S, Mohammed MA. Effect of pay-for-outcomes and encouraging new providers on National Health Service smoking cessation services in England: a cluster controlled study. PLoS One. 2015;10(4), e0123349.
5. Wallis MG, Lawrence G, Brenner RJ. Improving quality outcomes in a single-payer system: lessons learned from the UK National Health Service Breast Screening Programme. J Am Coll Radiol. 2008;5(6):737–43.
6. Hibbert P, Hannaford N, Long J, Plumb J, Braithwaite J. Final report: performance indicators used internationally to report publicly on healthcare organizations and local health systems. Australian Institute of Health Innovation, University of New South Wales; 2013.
7. Rosen B, Samuel H. Israel: health system review. World Health Organization. Health Systems in Transition, vol. 11, no. 2; 2009. http://www.euro.who.int/__data/assets/pdf_file/0007/85435/E92608.pdf. Accessed 2 Feb 2013.
8. Rosen B, Porath A, Pawlson LG, Chassin MR, Benbassat J. Adherence to standards of care by health maintenance organizations in Israel and the USA. Int J Qual Health Care. 2011;23(1):15–25.
9. Donzé JD, Williams MV, Robinson EJ, Zimlichman E, Aujesky D, Vasilevskis EE, Kripalani S, Metlay JP, Wallington T, Fletcher GS, Auerbach AD, Schnipper JL. International validity of the HOSPITAL score to predict 30-day potentially avoidable hospital readmissions. JAMA Intern Med. 2016;176(4):496–502.
10. Levi B, Borow M, Gelkin M. Participation of National Medical Associations in quality improvement activities—International comparison and the Israeli case. Israel J Health Policy Res. 2014;3:14
11. Pawlson GL. The evolving role of physician organizations in quality related activities. Israel J Health Policy Res. 2014;3:18.
12. Horowitz SD, Miller SH, Miles PV. Board certification and physician quality. Med Educ. 2004;38(1):10–1.
13. Brammli-Greenberg S, Gross R, Yair Y, Akiva E. Public opinion on the level of service and performance of the Healthcare System in 2009 and in comparison with previous years. 2011. Myers-JDC-Brookdale Institute. http://brookdale.jdc.org.il/?CategoryID=192&ArticleID=251. Accessed 15 April 2016.
14. Jaffe DH, Shmueli A, Ben-Yehuda A, Paltiel O, Calderon R, Cohen AD, Matz E, Rosenblum JK, Wilf-Miron R, Manor O. Community healthcare in Israel: quality indicators 2007–2009. Isreal J Health Policy Res. 2012;1(1):3.
15. Friedberg MW, Damberg CL. Methodological considerations in generating provider performance scores for use in public reporting: a guide for community quality collaborative. AHRQ. Pub 2011, No. 11-0093. Rockville: Agency for Healthcare Research and Quality.
16. Chassin MR. Quality of care: how good is good enough? Israel J Health Policy Res. 2012;1:4.
17. Jha AK, Perlin JB, Kizer KW, Dudley RA. Effect of the transformation of the Veterans Affairs Health Care System on the quality of care. N Engl J Med. 2003;348(22):2218–27.
18. Nirel N, Rosen B, Sharon A, Samuel H, Cohen AD. The impact of an integrated hospital-community medical information system on quality of care and medical service utilization in primary-care clinics. Inform Health Soc Care. 2011;36(2):63–74.
19. Crosson FJ. 21st-century health care—the case for integrated delivery systems. N Engl J Med. 2009;361(14):1324–5.
20. Kizer KW, Dudley RA. Extreme makeover: transformation of the Veterans Health Care System. Annu Rev Public Health. 2009;30:313–39.

Chapter 9
Leadership to Encourage and Sustain Performance

Monica Jain and Bruce L. Gewertz

Introduction

In today's healthcare environment, we are challenged to serve the needs of our patients while attempting to manage financial pressures, payment reform, an expanding number of technical innovations, and other transformational changes. To adapt, organizations must assemble and integrate the right tools, systems, and people. This process cannot be successful without leaders who are both technically and emotionally capable.

In this chapter, we will address some of the tools needed to meet these objectives, focusing on four key leadership competencies:

1. Aligning the organization's goals
2. Identifying necessary resources and structure
3. Properly incentivizing employees
4. Developing future and emerging leaders through coaching

Process of Aligning Goals

Creating a Vision

The essential tasks of leadership are to align the efforts of the organization, show people why they should work to build a better future, and motivate them to sustain their commitment to the larger purpose [1, 2]. These efforts are initiated by the

M. Jain, M.D. • B.L. Gewertz, M.D. (✉)
Department of Surgery, Cedars-Sinai Medical Center,
8700 Beverly Blvd., Suite 8215NT, Los Angeles, CA 90048, USA
e-mail: bruce.gewertz@cshs.org

© Springer International Publishing Switzerland 2017
H.C. Sax (ed.), *Measurement and Analysis in Transforming Healthcare Delivery*, DOI 10.1007/978-3-319-46222-6_9

development of a vision statement. A proper vision is framed by the interests of all of the people touched by the organization, i.e., patients, faculty, employees, and community, and not just the interests of the board or top executives [1]. The most critical aspect of this process is having a clear image of the desired state. As Steven Covey asserts, highly effective people "begin with the end in mind" [3].

Numerous healthcare leaders have advocated compartmentalizing a vision into key results areas that are all required for organizational excellence [4, 5]. Quint Studer, founder of the Studer Group, describes a "Five Pillar" model, consisting of Service, Quality, People, Finance, and Growth Pillars [4]. Likewise, Sharp, a large health system in San Diego, CA, promotes a "Seven Pillar" model, adding Safety and Community Pillars to Studer's model [6]. Regardless of the model used, key results areas provide a focus for organizational goals and maintain balance in terms of the short- and long-term objectives [4, 7, 8]. While each pillar is separate, the overarching vision aligns people and develops a sense of shared responsibility for the organization. Furthermore, the pillars are complementary, with success under one reaping rewards across each of the others [4].

Goal Setting

With a sound foundation based on a consensus vision, a leader can define organizational goals. This process begins with objective assessments of the current state. It is the gap between the current reality and the desired future that creates tension and the energy to move forward [8].

As a first step, it is wise to "throw caution to the wind and examine your patient." Leaders need to harness the collective insight of the frontline employees and the customers. These are the people who know where the system is broken and can help identify barriers to achieving the organization's vision. One method is to administer patient and employee satisfaction surveys. Unfortunately, these relatively simple tools usually do not reveal the full picture and often provide only superficial insights.

A more effective method of evaluating an organization is a concept commonly known as "managing by walking around" or "rounding for outcomes" [4, 7, 9]. By repeatedly touring the various hospital units, physician's clinics, research laboratories, and even the cafeteria, leaders can learn what is going on at the ground level of the organization—which individuals, departments, or systems are functioning at a high level and what can be done better. Rounding in this manner also allows leaders the opportunity to visibly recognize and reward movement toward the organization's goals and continuously reinforce the organization's vision into the employees at all levels.

Second, it is critical to obtain reliable data in each of the key results areas on a recurring basis. Useful benchmark data can include a wide range of measures, such as patient satisfaction scores, readmission rates, employee turnover, or operating income. Taken together, these measures are, in effect, the organization's vital signs as well as powerful tools to focus process improvement. These metrics support the establishment of specific targets for the organization and designate which individuals should rightly be held accountable for attaining these targets [1, 4].

Finally, leaders must dispassionately confront the organization's strengths, weaknesses, and barriers/challenges. While these assessments generally expose common issues, such as problems in communication and time management, they can also reveal varying perspectives on the state of the organization. Closing these gaps and bringing the organization's leadership into alignment is essential.

Once the current state is adequately defined, future goals can be determined. Discussions with many healthcare leaders have suggested that effective goals are (1) focused and understandable, (2) relevant, (3) measurable, and (4) time limited [1, 4, 10, 11]. Properly selected goals guide the processes put in place to achieve them and do not drain time, attention, and resources. Such goals provide focus and clarity to the organization's vision, bringing practicality to the organizational dream.

In our experience, there is a critical balance between the magnitude of the goal and the time projected for completion. The great architect and city planner of Chicago, Daniel Burnham (1846–1912) famously said, "Make no little plans, they have no magic to stir men's blood." Goals must be grand enough to inspire ascent to the "should be" state. Nonetheless, with short-term and modest goals as well as prolonged and substantial goals, employees often lose focus and ambition. Some may be discouraged, thinking either that their leaders do not have faith in them or that they may not have a long enough tenure to enjoy the outcome. By dividing large tasks into a series of important interim goals that are attainable, but not easily so, a greater motivation and sense of urgency is created. For example, if a medical center has a vision to establish a comprehensive cancer center, a venture that may require 5–10 years, it is useful to establish several specific interval targets, such as the establishment of a transdisciplinary research program, on the path to the eventual goal. Achievement of these steps will provide well-timed and positive reinforcements for the efforts.

Creating an Expectation of Success

Aligning an organization not only necessitates a definitive vision and set of goals but also requires sustained enthusiasm for the change process. Oftentimes, employees are motivated to change their behaviors only when the issues are so bad that they pose an existential threat. This produces temporary motivation that dies down as soon as the issues are less pressing [8].

Leaders are advantaged when followers consistently perform beyond expectations due to a sense of ownership [12, 13]. Such "transformational leadership" hardwires behaviors of excellence into employees and ingrains a culture of learning into the organization [7, 8, 10]. Studies of this leadership style have demonstrated that employees who understand the connection between their individual efforts and the overall goals of the organization are more engaged, focused, and productive [11].

At every level, communication is key to aligning an organization [1, 4, 7, 8, 14, 15]. For example, if a nurse does not understand that increased duration of urinary catheterization is strongly associated with risk of urinary tract infections (UTI), does not know the hospital's data regarding UTI rates and related patient outcomes, and is unaware of the Medicare policy that penalizes hospitals for catheter-associated UTI, he/she may find a hospital's directive to remind physicians to remove urinary catheters to be arbitrary or pointless; predictably, compliance with such a directive will be poor.

Communication also boosts employee morale. The healthcare industry is too often saddled with a culture in which only negative feedback occurs. When was the last time you heard of a nurse calling the laboratory to thank them for processing and delivering lab results in a timely fashion? As previously mentioned, the technique of rounding allows for positive feedback to numerous employees and departments, which improves attitudes and fosters optimism and determination. Additionally, by clearly communicating or displaying an organization's progress toward its goals, leaders are able to drive desired behaviors and align the organization toward the common goals.

As in every industry, healthcare leaders must be consistent, transparent, and genuine. By displaying external behaviors that are fully concordant with one's internal feelings and attitudes, leaders project positive behaviors and attitudes that permeate the organization [14]. Because unconscious emotions or intentions may drive emotions or behaviors, leaders must also take responsibility for their view of the world and not blame others for their personal issues [8, 15].

Today's dynamic and unpredictable healthcare environment demands adaptable organizations. The time has passed in which all solutions are "figured out at the top." Thus, healthcare leaders must enable employees by teaching them how to learn and how to think [8, 15]. This motivates people to not only leverage their collective genius to solve larger problems but also to get out of their comfort zones, learn new skills, and overcome any obstacles or resistance that they may encounter [1].

Identifying Necessary Resources and Structure

Identifying the discrepancies between "what is" and "what should be" is the critical step on the path to change. However, the necessary resources and structure to fill the gaps can be difficult to specify. Further, the collection of more and more data is rarely the solution.

The complex nature of the healthcare industry and the current movement toward collaborative teams requires a systems thinking approach to identifying necessary resources and structure. Systems thinking is the ability to recognize, understand, and synthesize the interactions and interdependencies in a set of components designed for a specific purpose [16]. Leaders thinking in this way can more easily identify the gaps and prioritize the proposed interventions [8].

One of the best methods in our experience involves "tests of change." In this process, those most closely involved with an activity are empowered to recommend and design interventions specifically targeted at fixing a problem. The implementation of these solutions (e.g., additional personnel, changes in protocols, spatial reorganization) is positioned as an experiment rather than as a permanent change. Moreover, the working teams objectively analyze each component for its intrinsic merit. Instead of a summative conclusion, a more nuanced view can be gained. Importantly, management can thereby demonstrate both receptiveness to feedback and flexibility in operations.

In such endeavors, the greatest resources by far are the frontline employees. Leaders need to pinpoint high performing people, units, or departments, and profile them to find out what it is that makes them successful. Leaders should also empower the employees to consider the overall needs and function of the organization. This bottom-up approach has the highest likelihood of unearthing the deficiencies within the organization and the obstacles to achieving the organizational goals. Under the best circumstances it engenders trust and buy-in, and further energizes people to work together to build a better future [1, 4].

As a practical example, Emergency Department length of stay data might demonstrate a long patient wait time, increasing patient dissatisfaction. Direct observation of and focused interviews with Emergency Department physicians and staff reveals that more patients could be seen and treated at any given time, but there are not enough beds in the Emergency Department to bring in more patients from the waiting room. Focus groups determine which incremental space, personnel, and supporting services are required. Finally, with a sense of the effects of these changes on the system, the costs/benefits of the needed investment are assessed, and the organization is able to institute an effective strategy to achieve its goals.

Incentives

It is generally accepted that "you get what you incent." Like most aphorisms, there is much truth in the statement. That being said, it is not always easy to know what the precise impact of a given incentive is on personal and group behaviors or what secondary consequences may ensue. Particularly in complex professional occupations in which there is considerable latitude for personal discretion, such as medicine, uncertainties regarding the effects of new incentives are common.

Good and Bad Consequences of Incentives

All would agree that organizations are entitled to expect dedicated service and professional achievement, and thus it would be wise to set up salary arrangements or reward systems that promote the same. Additionally, over the last decade, stressors such as down-trending reimbursements and increased scrutiny of outcomes have predictably amplified the attention paid to individual performance.

As a consequence, specific indicators of the volume and complexity of clinical work, such as wRVU's (work relative value units) have assumed a prominent place in the evaluation of physician productivity. In most modern clinical operations, wRVU targets are set for individual practitioners based on their allocation of clinical effort and the national norms for their specialty. Much effort is expended to parse out the percentage of effort for each component of their work and to ensure that their subspecialty norms are accounted for. In our experience, this process has substantial value in setting both individual and organizational expectations. Focusing on individual output and needed changes in effort, and then tying these more directly to compensation, has generally resulted in increased individual productivity in a variety of settings [17]. However, there are a number of adverse consequences of such measurements.

One weakness of this process is the tendency of practitioners to conclude that if some is good, more is better. This is particularly true in procedural specialties, in which the physicians are highly motivated, and the culture regards volume of work as a point of pride. The willingness to perform procedures is rarely the issue—when presented with volume targets, it is not uncommon for physicians to work well beyond rational expectations. With such high productivity, rewards are reaped across multiple organizational goals.

Nevertheless, more is not indeed better. Because of the emphasis on wRVUs, intragroup collaboration decreases, and section leaders tend to be wary of increasing manpower because of concerns over a "dilution" effect. Ultra-high caseloads are viewed as "insurance" against the loss of status or income. At a certain level of overwork, attention to detail can lag, and disruptive behavior becomes more frequent [18]. Other valued but less easily quantified behaviors, such as the appropriateness of treatments and patient satisfaction, may decline. Overall, the long-term success of the clinical unit can be compromised.

The Shortcomings of Individual Accountability

These observations highlight the second and perhaps most important limitation of using financial incentives to drive behavior. The major satisfier of high performing professionals is not compensation per se. While it may seem counterintuitive at first consideration, this seems to be true irrespective of the industry.

In his book "What Got You Here Won't Get You There," Marshall Goldsmith interviewed 200 "stars" from a wide variety of for-profit and non-profit organizations [19]. He was interested in understanding what factors predisposed to the retention of such high performers, considering that their success undoubtedly made them attractive to lucrative offers elsewhere. In these anonymous and detailed interviews with valued employees, he asked, "Why will you be here in 5 years?" He noted that the top three responses rarely included salary or bonuses. Rather, respondents frequently cited work and interpersonal factors—"I like the people I work with. I enjoy the work. The organization is giving me the chance to do what I want to do."

While straightforward on the surface, these simple answers reflect a highly nuanced blending of personal satisfaction and team goals. They suggest that for high performers, pride in individual achievement and positive group behaviors are the key motivators of outstanding work. The risk of discounting these drivers is not trivial.

The easiest and most direct adjustment is to modify productivity measures to include sectional or organizational targets in addition to individual targets. The weight given to group goals should increase as physicians become more senior, but even entry-level physicians should have some programmatic targets. In sum, the growth of the program as a whole needs to be made the highest priority for all practitioners.

Other Limitations of Financial Incentives

After adjusting bonus compensations in a number of procedural specialties to include programmatic targets, we observed a slower and less complete response than we anticipated. Case sharing and equalization of workload were more prevalent, but work imbalances, occasionally associated with noncollegial behaviors, were nonetheless persistent.

As noted by Marshall Goldsmith and by Brown and Gunderman, physician satisfaction and performance are closely tied to maximizing the time during which physicians perform the professional activities that they enjoy doing [20]. Taking this to a managerial level, cash bonuses must be combined with nonfinancial "intrinsic rewards" in order to be effective [21]. Organizations have approached this balance in a variety of ways: (1) adjusting the work schedules of physicians such that a more ideal distribution of research, clinical, and personal time can be achieved; or (2) providing additional resources (assistants, research support, etc.) that make their day-to-day lives more productive and enjoyable [22, 23].

Even considering the limitations, incentives and performance expectations are both useful and necessary. It is unquestioned that the financial benefit is always appreciated and is influential in sustaining motivation and retaining high performing practitioners. That said, there is considerable evidence that, irrespective of the industry, cash incentives are limited in their ability to reshape culture and organizational behavior. The misstep is overreliance on their power coupled with an illusion that fine-tuning incentives will be uniformly effective in modifying the behaviors of professionals.

Two additional lessons appear clear. First, after the initiation of any incentive program, it is important to objectively assess the true "downstream" effects and adjust appropriately. While too frequent modifications can be unsettling to all, maintaining an ineffective program more seriously undermines managerial credibility. Second, and most importantly, a great incentive program cannot act as a substitute for hiring and promoting the right people whose values parallel that of the organization as a whole.

Coaching

Atul Gawande's compelling article entitled "Personal Best" emphasizes the importance of lifelong development and coaching. He asserts that "no matter how well prepared people are in their formative years, few can achieve and maintain their best performance on their own" [24]. Unfortunately, he also points out how infrequently medical professionals are observed and coached. For example, surgeons train for 5–7 years

under the vigilant gaze and continuous instruction of senior practitioners. After gradua-
tion from residency/fellowship, it is assumed that they no longer need instruction, and
they perform procedures essentially unobserved for 40 years. A similar narrative often
plays out in medical management as well. High performers are promoted to supervisory
positions for extraordinary clinical skills and are expected to spontaneously develop the
full range of leadership capabilities. In case of failure, corrective actions are deferred to
avoid upsetting a critical producer and the efficacy of leadership flounders.

The capacity for leadership can be expanded by a number of methods, including
coursework, the thoughtful observation of good and bad examples, and personal
experience. Still, insightful executives soon realize that they would profit from an
independent evaluator who helps them see both their environment and their own
actions more clearly.

The challenges to successful leadership development in medical environments are
actually not substantially different from other professions with driven and highly competent people. The acceptance of coaching is strongly influenced by the culture of the
organization, and medicine historically lacks any structured mentoring programs. This
may be a result of the ambiguity with which many physicians view leadership and
management functions [25]. If mid-level executives are aware that their superiors
engage in similar self-improvement activities, it becomes clear that coaching is a wise
investment in an individual, rather than an isolated punitive or corrective action.

Initiating a "therapeutic" coaching relationship is also a delicate matter. Phil
Jackson, one of the most successful professional basketball coaches of all time,
always emphasized to his players that irrespective of their tenure on his team, his
promise to them was to develop their personal skills and enhance their overall value.
This commitment motivated them even if their role on the team was not large [14].
A mentee must be motivated and open to change. Enthusiasm for coaching is greatest after "teachable moments," when circumstances make it clear to the subject that
modifications in behaviors are needed. This could occur at the time of promotion or
when an important adaptive challenge is identified. The coaching relationship also
necessitates a thoughtful match between coach and mentee. For some, the best
choice is a coach with common history and personality (i.e., of the same specialty
or following a similar career path). Others profit most from a true outsider, whose
experiences may even be in a different industry.

In short, as the need for teamwork and collaboration between physicians, other
caregivers, and administration becomes more evident in today's healthcare environment, we can expect professional coaching and leadership development to be
viewed as one of the most important corporate assets.

Conclusion

Effective leadership that initiates and maintains high levels of performance at multiple levels of an organization is a challenge, irrespective of the industry. To further
the discussion, we have shared some of our personal experiences and the thoughtful

insights of others. Above all, it is unquestioned that sustaining excellence requires extraordinary attention to the entire work environment along with the highest level of interpersonal skills.

References

1. Souba WW. The new leader: new demands in a changing, turbulent environment. J Am Coll Surg. 2003;197(1):79–87.
2. Drath WH. Leading together: complex challenges require a new approach. Leadersh Action. 2003;23(1):3–7.
3. Covey SR. The 7 habits of highly effective people. New York: Free Press; 2004.
4. Studer Q. Hardwiring excellence. Gulf Breeze: Fire Starter Publishing; 2003.
5. Sherman VC. Creating the New American Hospital: a time for greatness. San Francisco: Jossey-Bass; 1993.
6. Pillars of Excellence. The sharp experience. 2016. http://www.sharp.com/about/the-sharp-experience/pillars-excellence.cfm.
7. Studer Q, Straight A. Leadership. Gulf Breeze: Fire Starter Publishing; 2009.
8. Senge PM. The leader's new work: building learning organizations. MIT Sloan Management Review. 1990.
9. Ridky J, Sheldon GF. Managing in academics: a health center model. St. Louis: Quality Medical Publishing; 1993.
10. Copeland III EM. Lessons learned as a surgical chairman. Am Surg. 2002;68(6):505–7.
11. Kotter JP. What leaders really do. Harvard Business review on leadership. Boston: Harvard Business School Publishing; 1998.
12. Scully NJ. Leadership in nursing: the importance of recognising inherent values and attributes to secure a positive future for the profession. Collegian. 2015;22(4):439–44.
13. Kapu AN, Jones P. APRN transformational leadership. Nurs Manage. 2016;47:19–22.
14. Gewertz BL, Logan DC. The best medicine. New York: Springer; 2015.
15. Ludeman K, Erlandson E. Radical change, radical results. Chicago: Dearborn Trade Publishing; 2003.
16. Phillips JM, Stalter AM, Dolansky MA, Lopez GM. Fostering future leadership in quality and safety in health care through systems thinking. J Prof Nurs. 2016;32(1):15–24.
17. Brown R, Cabral J. Moving the dial with employee and executive incentives. Leadership. 2013.
18. Shanafelt TD, Boone S, Tan L, Dyrbye LN, Sotile W, Satele D, West CP, Sloan J, Oreskovich MR. Burnout and satisfaction with work-life balance among US physicians relative to the general US population. Arch Intern Med. 2012;172(18):1377–85.
19. Goldsmith M, Reiter M. What got you here won't get you there. New York: Hyperion; 2007.
20. Brown S, Gunderman RB. Viewpoint: enhancing the professional fulfillment of physicians. Acad Med. 2006;81:577–82.
21. Herzberg F. One more time: how do you motivate employees? Harv Bus Rev. 2003;81(1):87–96.
22. Cahn ES, Gray C. The time bank solution. Stanford Social Innovation Review; 2015.
23. Schulte B. Time in the bank: a Stanford plan to save doctors from burnout. The Washington Post. 2015.
24. Gawande A. Personal best: top athletes and singers have coaches. Should you? The New Yorker: Conde Nast; 2011.
25. Fairbain P. Personal communication from E. Trist. In: Gilmore TN, editor. Challenges for physicians in formal leadership roles. Philadelphia: Center for Applied Research; 2002.

Index

© Springer International Publishing Switzerland 2017   123
H.C. Sax (ed.), *Measurement and Analysis in Transforming Healthcare
Delivery*, DOI 10.1007/978-3-319-46222-6

The manufacturer's authorised representative in the EU is Springer
Nature Customer Service Centre GmbH, Europaplatz 3, 69115 Heidelberg,
Germany. If you have any concerns regarding our products, please
contact ProductSafety@springernature.com

Printed and bound by CPI Group (UK) Ltd, Croydon, CR0 4YY
11/05/2026
02107196-0001